QUESTIONS AND ANSWERS

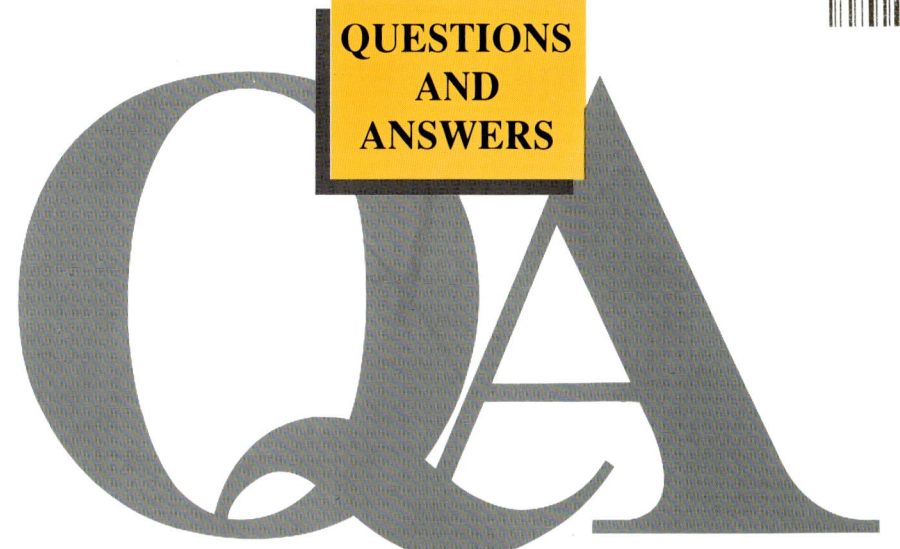

THE HUMAN BODY

Text: Gillian Bunce
Illustrations: Ian Lusted
Consultants: Dr Philip Segar and Dr Chris Warton

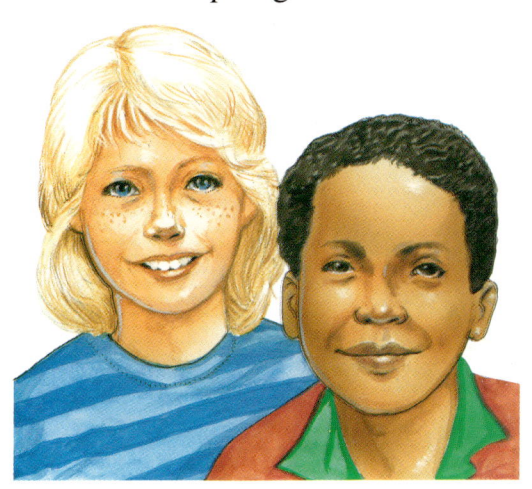

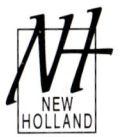

NEW
HOLLAND

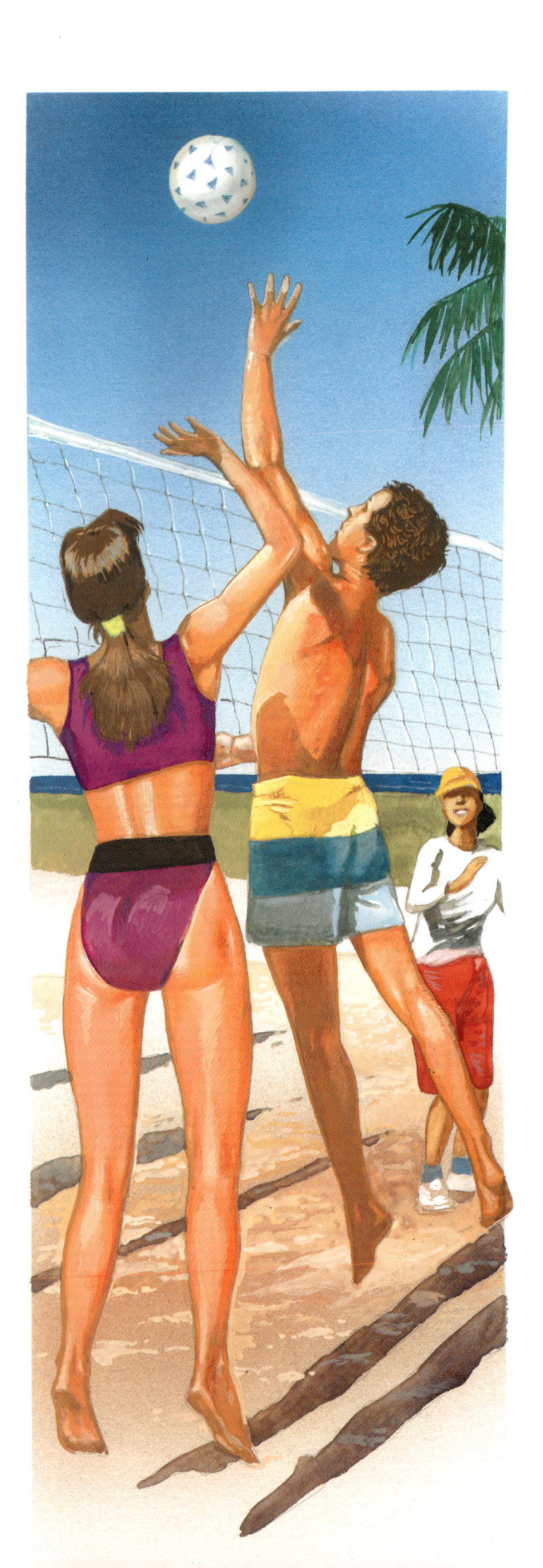

Contents

First published in the UK in 1994 by
New Holland (Publishers) Ltd
24 Nutford Place, London W1H 6DQ

Reprinted in 1995

ISBN 1 85368 355 8

Editor: Sean Fraser
Designer: Tracey Carstens
Illustrations: Ian Lusted

Typeset by Suzanne Fortescue, Struik DTP
Reproduction by Unifoto (Pty) Ltd
Printed and bound in Singapore by Kyodo Printing Co (Pte) Ltd

Introduction

Your body is your most valuable possession, but many people probably don't think of it that way. The human body contains many organs and, although each has its own job, the organs also work together to carry out important functions. At any moment of the day or night, there are many things are happening inside you. Your heart is pumping blood through your arteries and veins. Your lungs are drawing air in and out. Your kidneys are removing waste. Electric signals are flashing along your nerves. Damaged cells are repairing themselves. Your blood cells are fighting germs. All these activities, and many, many more, take place all the time and give you the precious gift of life.

Can you name these parts of your body? The answers are on page 32.

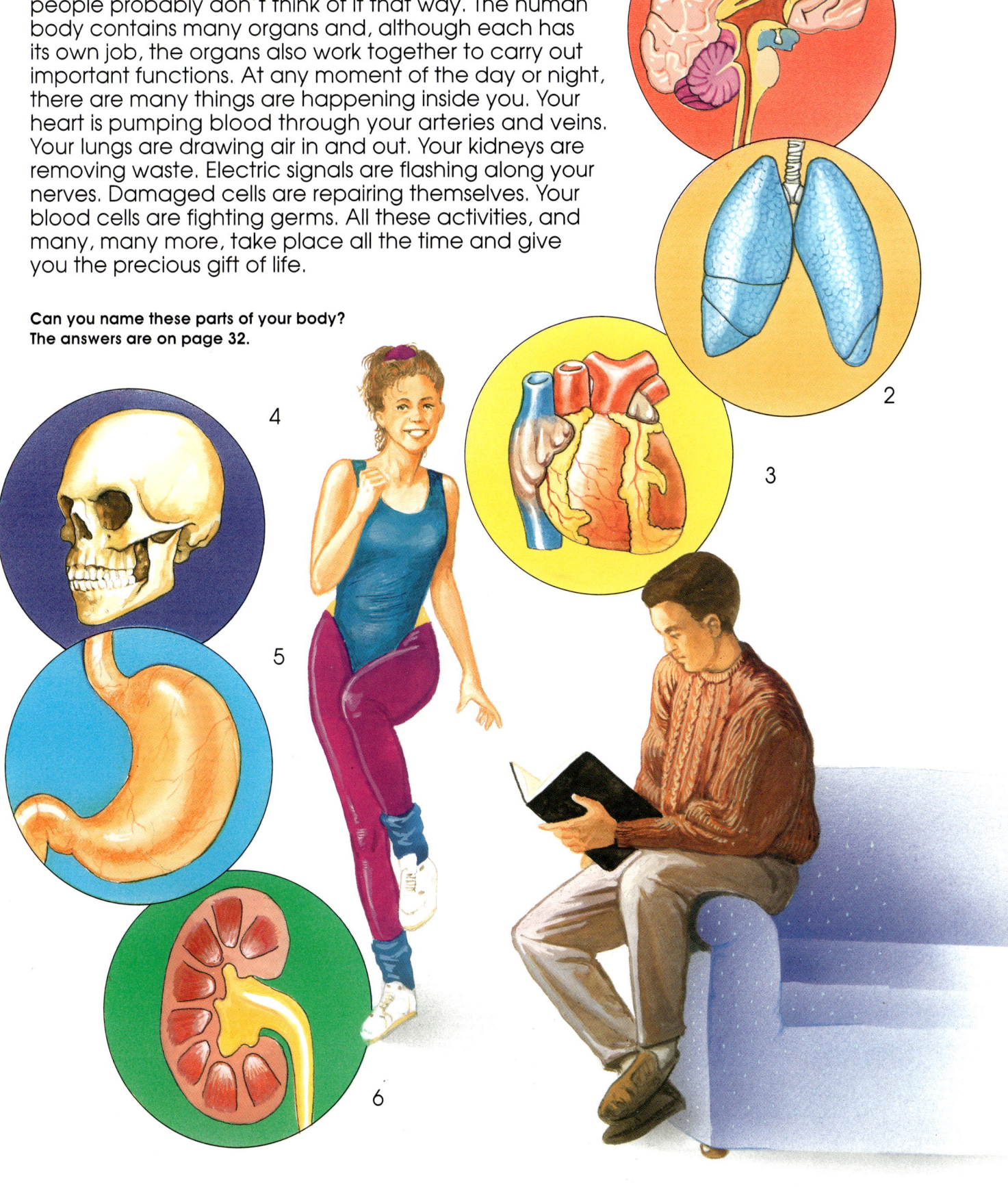

Your body's building blocks

Your body is like a large city with many different factories, only much more efficient. It is made up of many smaller parts, each with a different job. The smallest living parts of your body, the cells, are like tiny factories that work day and night to keep you alive.

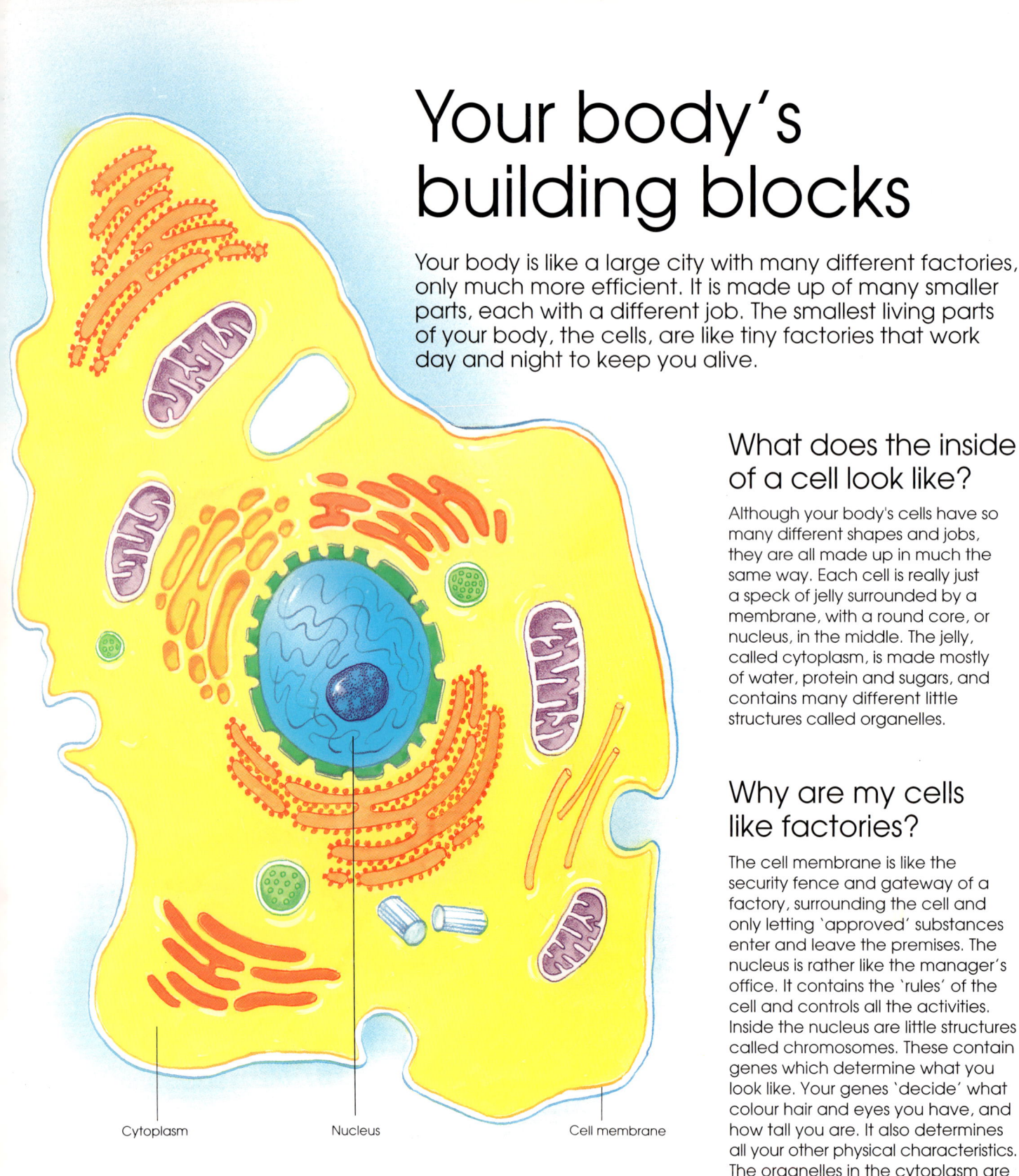

Cytoplasm   Nucleus   Cell membrane

What are the ingredients of my body?

The elements that make up your body are so basic that they are even found in the dry dust of the earth. The reason you are a growing, moving, eating, talking, thinking, living being, is the remarkable way these elements are put together in your body to make other substances. Between 70 and 85 per cent of your body is made of water. Some of the other important 'ingredients' are protein and carbohydrates.

What does the inside of a cell look like?

Although your body's cells have so many different shapes and jobs, they are all made up in much the same way. Each cell is really just a speck of jelly surrounded by a membrane, with a round core, or nucleus, in the middle. The jelly, called cytoplasm, is made mostly of water, protein and sugars, and contains many different little structures called organelles.

Why are my cells like factories?

The cell membrane is like the security fence and gateway of a factory, surrounding the cell and only letting 'approved' substances enter and leave the premises. The nucleus is rather like the manager's office. It contains the 'rules' of the cell and controls all the activities. Inside the nucleus are little structures called chromosomes. These contain genes which determine what you look like. Your genes 'decide' what colour hair and eyes you have, and how tall you are. It also determines all your other physical characteristics. The organelles in the cytoplasm are like the factory's workers, doing many different jobs: they prepare raw materials such as food to be used in the cell, 'offload' energy from food, make new protein and store it, 'package' goods to be delivered to other cells, and get rid of waste products.

Could I count the cells in my body?

No. There are billions – and more than 100 different kinds. Apart from the female egg cell (see page 31), cells are too small to be seen with the naked eye. And although nerve cells are very long (see page 18), they are still too thin to be seen. Each cell has its own special job. It receives oxygen from the air you breathe and nutrients from the food you eat, and changes them into other chemical substances which your body needs. As the cell does this it gives off heat and energy which keeps it going.

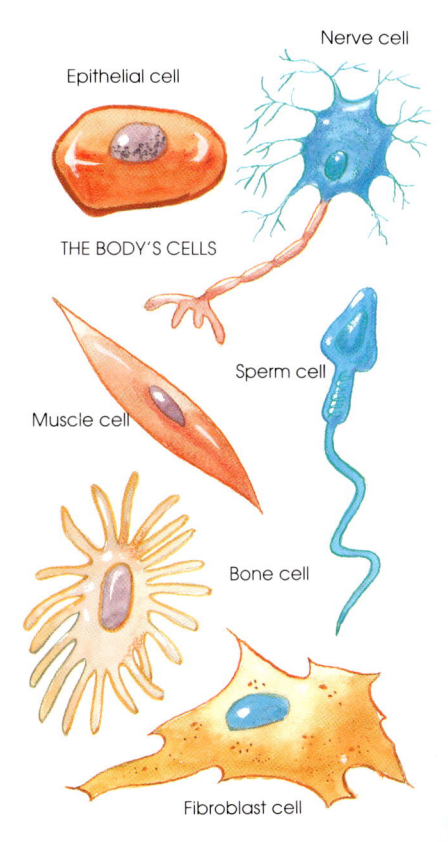

Epithelial cell

Nerve cell

THE BODY'S CELLS

Muscle cell

Sperm cell

Bone cell

Fibroblast cell

Is there a 'zoo' inside me?

Of course not. But if you look at a drawing of the many different kinds and shapes of your body cells it is easy to imagine them as little animals. Nerve cells, for example, look like octopuses. Sperm cells look like tadpoles. The cells of your skin fit together rather like honeycomb – as though a bee had made them. Your bone cells look a bit like spider webs. There are also many other wonderful shapes: balls, buttons, boxes, cubes, cylinders, saucers and curls.

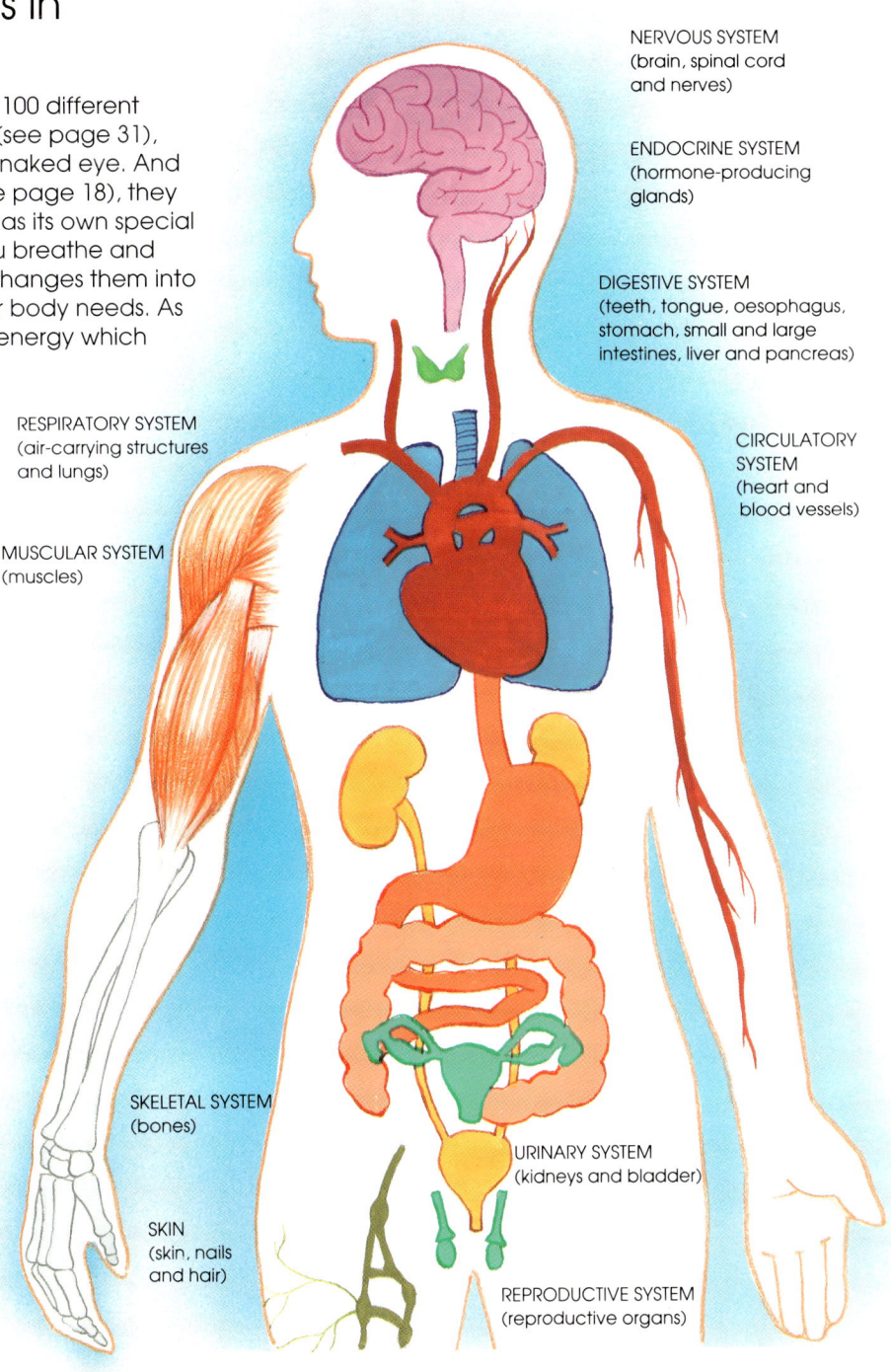

NERVOUS SYSTEM
(brain, spinal cord
and nerves)

ENDOCRINE SYSTEM
(hormone-producing
glands)

DIGESTIVE SYSTEM
(teeth, tongue, oesophagus,
stomach, small and large
intestines, liver and pancreas)

RESPIRATORY SYSTEM
(air-carrying structures
and lungs)

CIRCULATORY
SYSTEM
(heart and
blood vessels)

MUSCULAR SYSTEM
(muscles)

SKELETAL SYSTEM
(bones)

URINARY SYSTEM
(kidneys and bladder)

SKIN
(skin, nails
and hair)

REPRODUCTIVE SYSTEM
(reproductive organs)

Is my body just a jumble of cells?

No. Your cells are arranged in a special way in your body. Cells that look alike and do the same work are joined together to form tissue. Your muscle cells, for example, form muscle tissue. Tissues, in turn, are joined together to form organs. A muscle is an organ made up mostly of muscle tissue. Your organs, also work together to form a system. Your brain, spinal cord and the nerves running through your body, for example, form your nervous system. You have many different systems in your body. They do not work on their own, but help one another. When you exercise, for example, your muscles need more oxygen. So your respiratory system helps by taking in more oxygen.

Your framework

When an engineer designs a building or a bridge, he first plans a strong framework of steel beams. Your skeleton is like a remarkable system of beams strong enough to support all your flesh and organs.

Why do I need a skeleton?

Your skeleton does a number of very useful things for you. Your bones give support and shape to your body. Without them, you would be as floppy as a jellyfish. They form an anchor to which your muscles are attached. Your bones help protect the organs of your body. The marrow inside your bones acts like a factory where blood cells are made. Lastly, your bones act like a pantry for storing minerals such as calcium.

How many bones are there in my body?

The number of bones changes as you grow. Some bones separate and others grow together (fuse). A baby is born with about 270 separate bones. A young teenager has about 350 bones. By the time you reach the age of 20 to 25 there are about 206 separate bones in your body. Two of the most important kinds of bones in your body are long bones, found in your arms, legs, fingers and toes, and flat bones, found in your skull. More than half your bones are in your hands, wrists, feet and ankles.

Can my funny bone really make me laugh?

No. The sensation blamed on your 'funny bone' is painful and unlikely to make you laugh. Your funny bone is not a bone at all, but a nerve passing your elbow, and is easily hurt. It lies next to the upper arm bone called the humerus which may be why we call it a funny bone.

SKELETON

Did you know?

Bones need the pressure they get from exercise. If you do not move, your bones lose calcium which makes them soft and fragile. The astronauts on early space missions lost a lot of calcium from their bones because the weightlessness of space put no pressure on their bones. Today astronauts follow exercise programmes in space to avoid this problem.

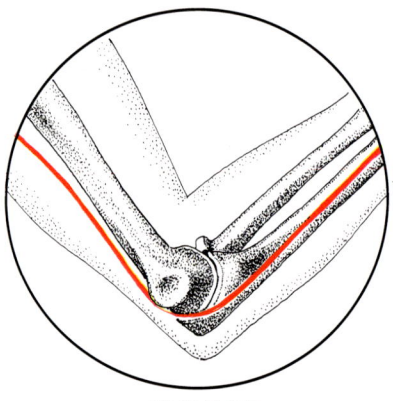

FUNNY BONE

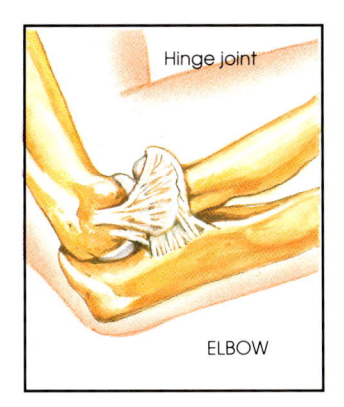

Hinge joint

ELBOW

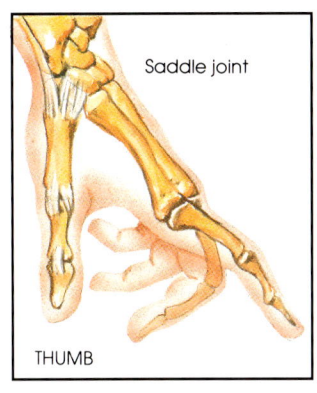

Saddle joint

THUMB

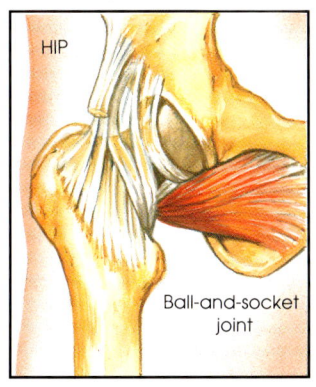

HIP

Ball-and-socket joint

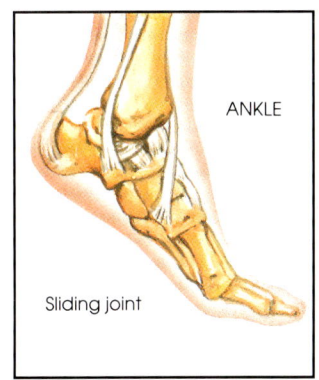

ANKLE

Sliding joint

Could my skeleton fall apart?

No, your bones are joined to one another at places called joints. Joints allow your muscles to move your bones into thousands of different positions. You have many different kinds of joints. Hinge joints are found in your elbows and knees and let you swing your arms and legs forwards and backwards. Ball-and-socket joints are found in your shoulders and hips. The round end of one bone fits snugly inside the hollow of the other, letting you twist and turn your arms and legs in almost any direction. Fibrous joints are found in your skull and do not allow any movement at all.

What keeps my joints 'joined'?

Your joints are held in place by bands of strong tissue called ligaments which stretch from one bone to another. Many of your joints are surrounded by a tube of tissue which also helps keep your bone ends together. It contains a liquid which 'oils' your bone ends and helps them slide smoothly over each other. The ends of your bones are covered by a layer of slippery, rubbery tissue called cartilage which helps your joints glide smoothly over one another and cushions the ends of your bones.

Are my bones really bone-dry?

The word 'skeleton' comes from a Greek word meaning dry, but the bones of your skeleton are not at all dry. In fact, about a third of bone is made up of water. The solid part of bone is made of three things: cells called osteocytes, minerals such as calcium and phosphorus, which make bone hard, and collagen, a special protein which gives bone its strength.

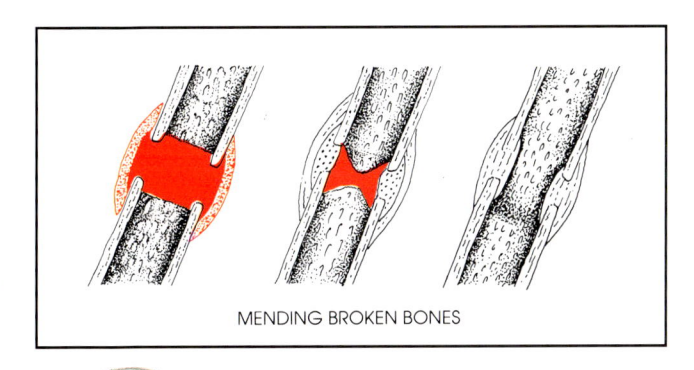

MENDING BROKEN BONES

Are my bones really hollow?

Yes. Even though a bone is filled with bone marrow, it is really just like a long, hollow tube, and only the knob on each end of the bone is solid. There are two types of bone tissue: compact bone, which is solid and smooth, and cancellous bone, which is spongy and lighter than compact bone. The shaft is made of mainly compact bone. The knob on either end of the bone consists of cancellous bone surrounded by compact bone. The outside of the bone is covered by a thin layer called the periosteum. Many nerves and blood vessels pass through the periosteum to the bone underneath.

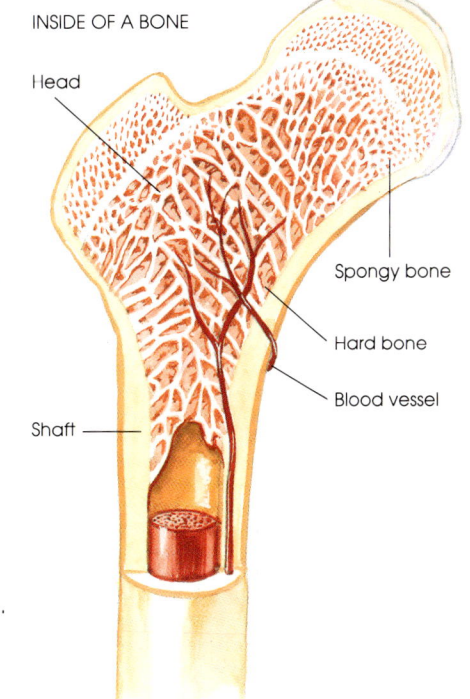

INSIDE OF A BONE

Head

Spongy bone

Hard bone

Blood vessel

Shaft

How does a broken bone heal?

A broken bone is called a fracture. When a bone breaks, the cells around the broken part produce a mass of cartilage and collagen (a type of protein) called a callus. The callus is gradually replaced by bone cells, and the bone heals. There are two main types of fractures. A simple fracture occurs when the bone breaks but does not pierce the skin. When the bone does pierce the skin this is called a compound fracture. A greenstick fracture occurs when a bone bends but does not break completely. These fractures are common in children because their bones are still quite soft.

On the move

When you eat a steak, you are actually eating a cow's muscle. Muscles are found everywhere in your body and form your flesh. They are usually attached to your bones and allow you to smile, to frown, to sit still, to play sport, to breathe and to digest food.

What happens when I bend my knee?

Although muscles do so many different things, they all move in only two ways: by contracting and relaxing. When your muscles contract, they become shorter and thicker. When they relax, they go back to their original size. Once a muscle has contracted, it has to be pulled back to its original size either by gravity or by another muscle. For this reason many muscles work in pairs, with each muscle in the pair pulling in the opposite direction. For example, the muscle at the back of your leg bends your knee and the one in front pulls it straight. Because muscles can only pull something to move it, both ends of the muscle must be attached to something firm, usually bone. Many muscles are anchored to bone by tough, thin cords of tissue called tendons.

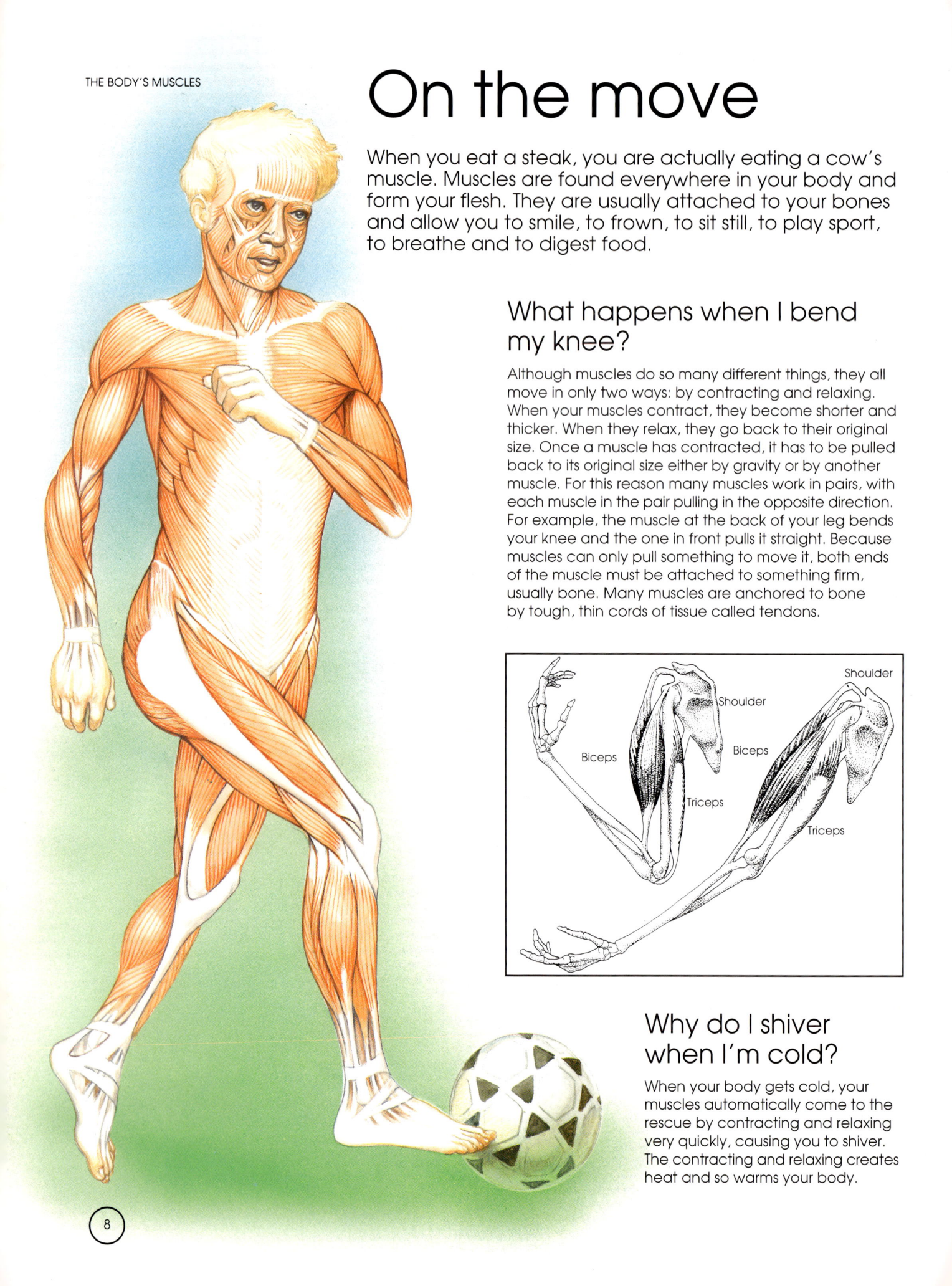

Why do I shiver when I'm cold?

When your body gets cold, your muscles automatically come to the rescue by contracting and relaxing very quickly, causing you to shiver. The contracting and relaxing creates heat and so warms your body.

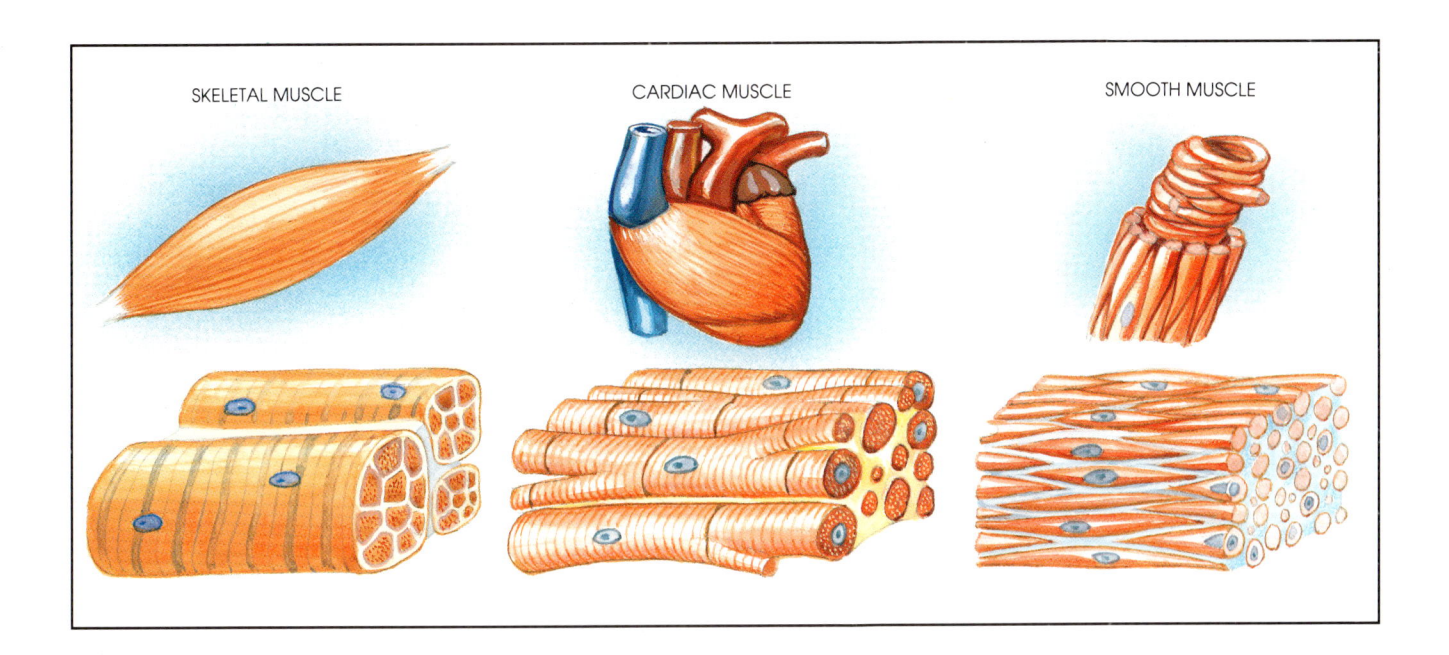

SKELETAL MUSCLE   CARDIAC MUSCLE   SMOOTH MUSCLE

Are all my muscles the same?

No. You have three kinds. Striped or striated muscle – named for its stripey appearance under the microscope – is the muscle that moves your bones, allowing you to do things like walk, chew, shake someone's hand and dance. Because you can control this muscle, it is described as voluntary. You have about 600 voluntary muscles in your body. Smooth muscle – so named because it does not have any stripes – lies in the walls of hollow organs like your blood vessels, digestive canal and bladder. It works automatically and so is called involuntary muscle. Heart or cardiac muscle makes up the walls of the heart. It is a special, involuntary muscle and looks stripey.

What does the inside of a muscle look like?

If you cut through a striped muscle you would find that it is made up of several thick bundles. Each bundle consists of muscle fibres. The fibres are long and cylindrical, and stretch down the length of the muscle. There can be as many as a quarter of a million fibres in one bundle. The fibres are made up of even smaller muscle fibrils.

Why do I sometimes get a stitch when I exercise?

When you exercise without allowing your body to warm up properly, your diaphragm (see page 12) suddenly has to work harder and can contract too tightly. The result is a painful cramp, which we call a stitch. You can also get cramps in many other muscles. Swimmer's cramp, a cramp in the muscles of the abdomen, is brought on when you suddenly get into cold water. Writer's cramp is caused when the muscles in your hand and fingers have been tightened for too long.

Do my muscles sleep when I do?

Most of your body's muscles become tired after a hard day's work or after exercise. They relax when you are asleep, although not completely, so your muscles are always slightly contracted. Scientists call this muscle tone. Muscle tone is one of the ways your body keeps warm. One important muscle that never tires in a healthy person is the heart. Your heart carries on beating, no matter how tired all your other muscles are.

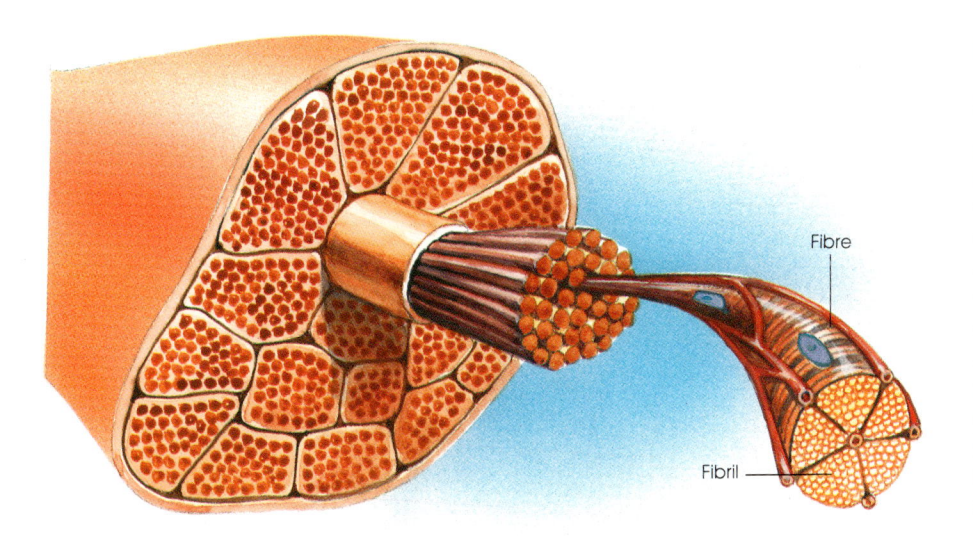

Fibre

Fibril

From the heart

Have you ever felt your heart beating in your chest? Day in and day out, this remarkable double pump contracts and relaxes, sending your blood on a never-ending journey through your body.

THE HEART

Left atrium

Left ventricle

Right atrium

Right ventricle

Is my heart really heart-shaped?

No. Your heart looks only roughly like the simple, red heart we often see on St Valentine's Day. Your heart is shaped more like an upside down pear. It is a muscular bag which consists of two separate pumps, one on the right and one on the left, and separated from each other by a wall of muscle called the septum. Each pump has two chambers. The top chamber is called the atrium and the bottom chamber the ventricle. Little flaps called valves lie at the exit of each chamber to make sure the blood flows in one direction only.

Is my heart on my left side?

Not really. Your heart lies near the middle of your chest, just a bit more to the left than to the right. It is slightly tilted, with its wide top part pointing to the right and its narrow bottom part pointing left and forwards. This is why you feel your heart thumping on the left.

POSITION OF THE HEART

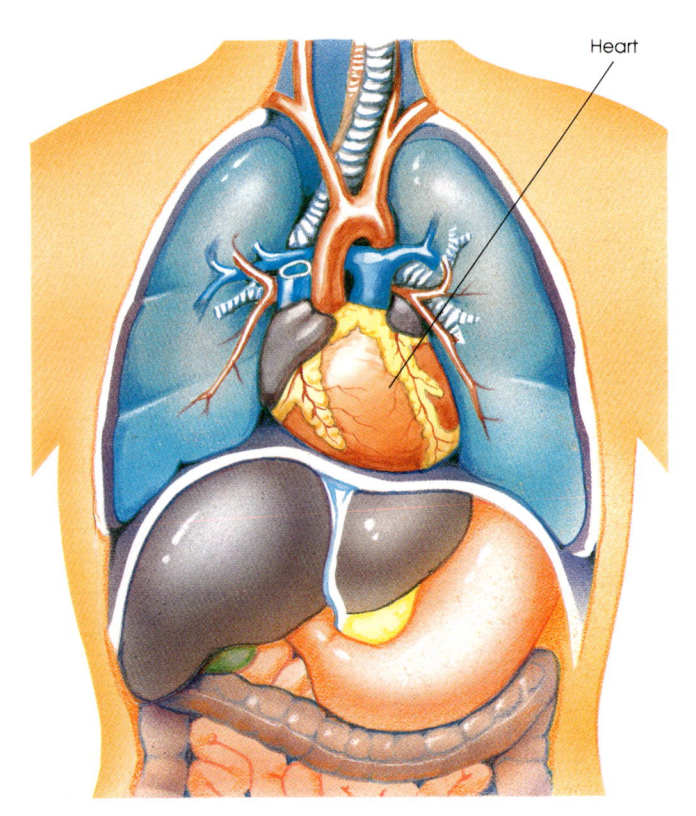

Heart

Do hearts really murmur?

Yes, most heart murmurs are low, rumbling sounds. But they may also be gentle hisses or roars. Some are quite harmless. They are simply the sounds of the blood moving through the heart. But sometimes a heart murmur means that there is something wrong with one of the heart valves. The sound may be caused by blood leaking back into one of the chambers. Doctors can usually repair faulty heart valves with surgery.

Why does my heart beat faster when I'm frightened?

When you are frightened, special glands above your kidneys send a hormone called adrenalin surging through your bloodstream. Adrenalin has a number of effects on your body, one of which is to make your heart beat faster. This causes more oxygen to reach your muscles and prepares you to deal with whatever is frightening you – perhaps by running away.

Are there really tunnels running into my heart?

Yes, your heart has tubes called blood vessels leading into and out of it. In fact, nearly every part of your body has blood vessels. The vessels that carry blood from your heart to your lungs and the different parts of your body are called arteries. Those that take blood from your body back to your heart are called veins.

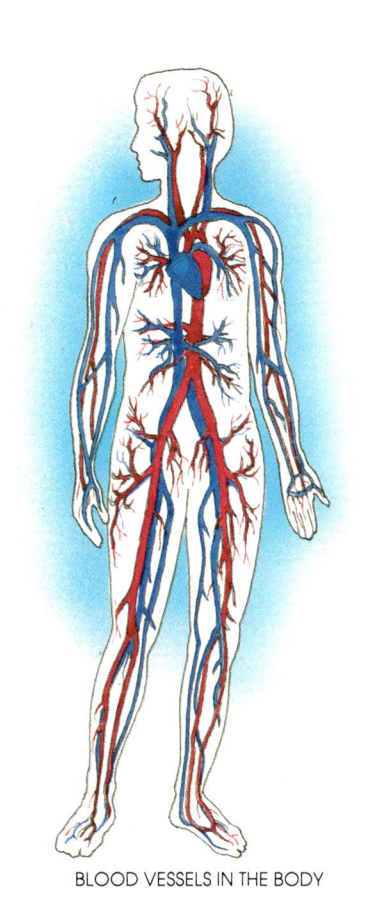

BLOOD VESSELS IN THE BODY

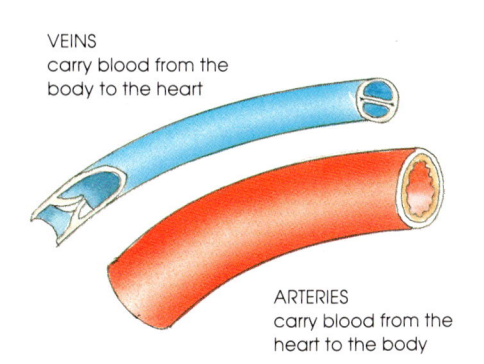

VEINS
carry blood from the body to the heart

ARTERIES
carry blood from the heart to the body

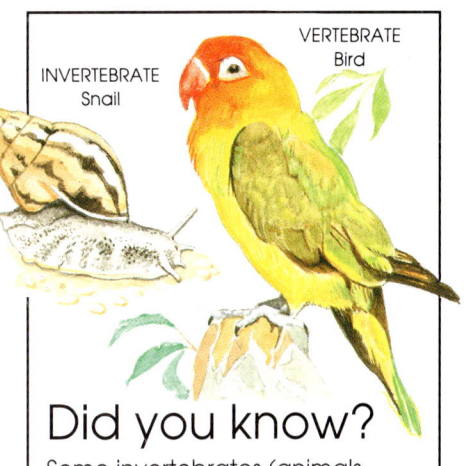

INVERTEBRATE
Snail

VERTEBRATE
Bird

Did you know?

Some invertebrates (animals without a backbone) such as earthworms, snails and flies have a heart, although they are much simpler than the human heart. All vertebrates (animals with a back-bone) such as fish, amphibians, reptiles, birds and mammals have a heart, which works much the same way as our's does.

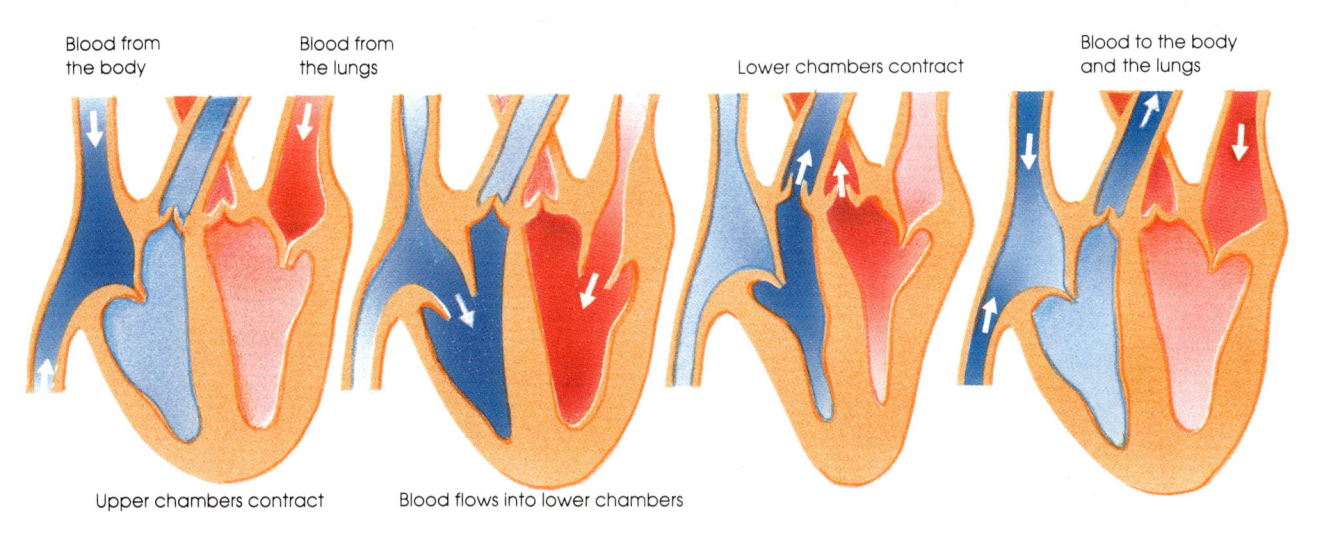

Blood from the body

Blood from the lungs

Lower chambers contract

Blood to the body and the lungs

Upper chambers contract

Blood flows into lower chambers

What makes my heart beat?

In the right atrium of your heart is some very special tissue. This tissue produces an electric current that makes the muscles of the two top chambers (or atria) contract. Within a fraction of a second the electrical current passes through to the bottom two chambers (or ventricles), which makes them contract. You feel these contractions as heartbeats.

Why does my heart have two separate pumps?

It would be a waste if oxygen-rich blood were to mix with blood which has very little oxygen. To avoid this, each pump deals with different blood – the right side with blood lacking in oxygen, the left side with oxygen-rich blood. When blood fills your right atrium, the muscle of that chamber contracts and forces the blood through the valve into the right ventricle. When the right ventricle fills with blood, the muscle of that chamber contracts and pushes the blood through a valve into an artery leading to your lungs. The left side of your heart works in the same way. Blood is squeezed from the left atrium into the left ventricle, and then leaves the heart in an artery which carries it to the rest of your body.

Breath of life

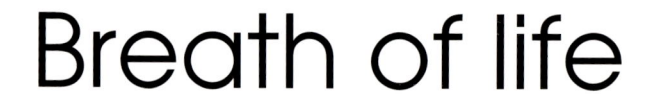

Just as cars need petrol, and trains coal or electricity, the human body needs fuel to burn up to create energy for its life processes. This fuel comes from the nutrients in the food we eat and oxygen in the air we breathe. The human respiratory system not only transports life-giving oxygen from the atmosphere to the cells in our bodies, but helps rid the body of waste products too.

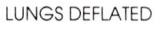

RIB CAGE

Are my lungs in a cage?

Yes, a cage of bone. Your two lungs are inside your chest, one on either side. They are protected by your ribs, spine and breastbone which, together with the rib muscles, form a 'cage' around them. Also in this cage are your heart, some blood vessels, oesophagus and windpipe. The right lung is divided into three parts called lobes and is slightly larger than the left lung, which has only two lobes, because it has to share space with the heart. The lungs are protected at the bottom by a sheet of muscle called the diaphragm.

What is sneezing, coughing and hiccuping?

Sneezing occurs when the mucous membranes of your nose are irritated by particles of dust, pollen or germs. First you breathe in, and then the air is forced violently from your lungs through your mouth and nose, blasting out the irritating particles. Coughing is a bit like sneezing, except that the irritating particles lie lower down in your respiratory system – around your voice box, trachea or bronchi. Hiccuping can result from eating or drinking too much or too quickly. When you get the hiccups your diaphragm contracts and you breathe in very quickly. As this happens, the space between your vocal cords suddenly closes, causing the typical clicking sound.

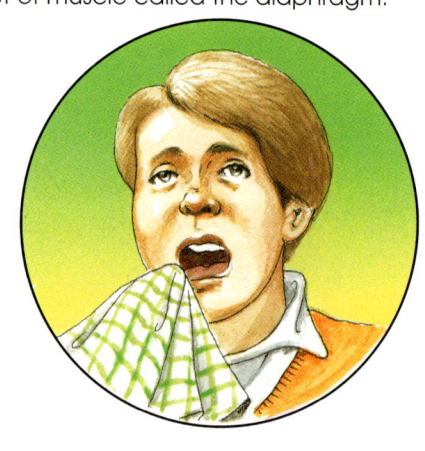

LUNGS DEFLATED

LUNGS INFLATED

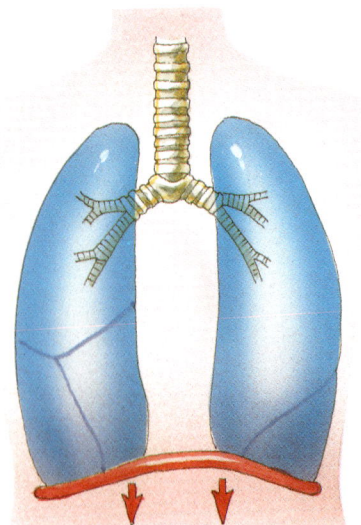

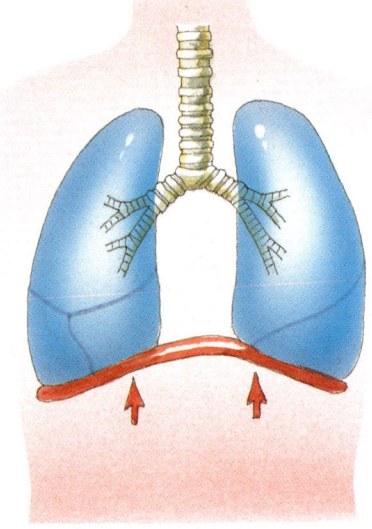

DIAPHRAGM RELAXED

DIAPHRAGM CONTRACTED

How does air get into my lungs?

The flow of air in and out of your lungs is caused by the tightening and relaxation of mainly the diaphragm and the rib muscles. When you breathe in, your diaphragm moves down and your ribs move outwards. Your lungs expand and air rushes in. When you breathe out again, your diaphragm relaxes and your ribs return to their normal position. Your lungs contract so air is forced out. Membranes covering the lungs and inside the chest wall allow the lungs to move freely as you breathe.

How do my lungs work?

Air enters your body through your nose and mouth and then passes through the throat and voice box to your windpipe, or trachea. The trachea divides into two branches, called the bronchi, each of which leads into a lung. Once inside the lungs, the bronchi divide rather like the branches of a tree and form smaller and smaller branches until they form tiny tubes which are called bronchioles. The bronchioles end in tiny sacs called alveoli. The walls of the alveoli contain thousands of tiny blood capillaries. It is inside the alveoli that gases interchange between the air and the blood. Oxygen passes through the walls of the alveoli into the blood in the capillaries. Some of the oxygen dissolves in the blood, but most combines with haemoglobin (see page 14) and is then transported to the tissues of your body. At the same time that oxygen passes into the blood, carbon dioxide, a waste gas, leaves the blood and is eventually breathed out.

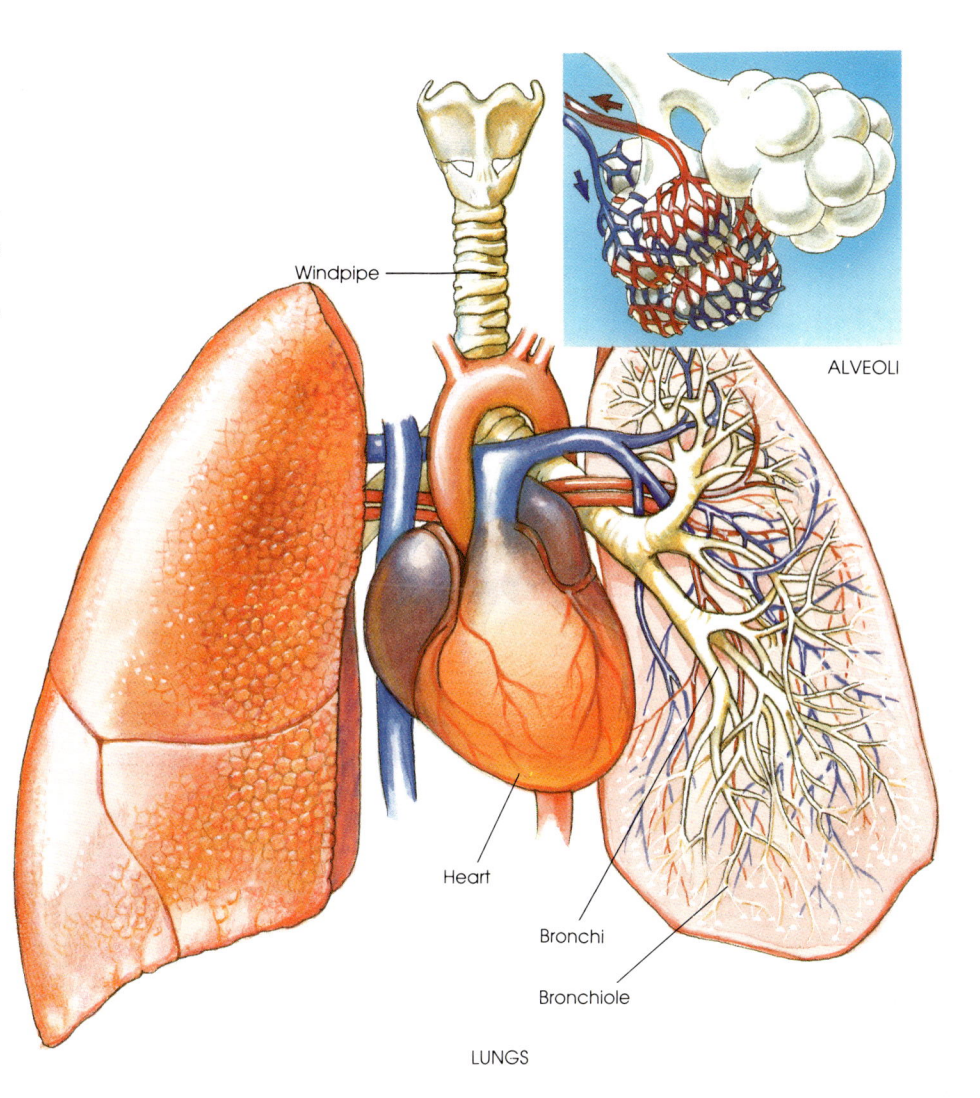

ALVEOLI

Windpipe

Heart

Bronchi

Bronchiole

LUNGS

How does smoking damage the lungs?

Smoking cigarettes stops the lungs from doing their job properly, and can lead to serious illnesses such as lung cancer, emphysema and heart disease. The smoke from burning tobacco contains many poisonous gases, among them carbon monoxide, nicotine and tars. These poisons cause the lungs to make lots of slimy mucus. The poisons also damage the little hairs that line the air passages and stop them from doing their job of wafting dust and other foreign matter away. This is why smokers cough. Over long periods the poisons damage the cells and may cause cancer.

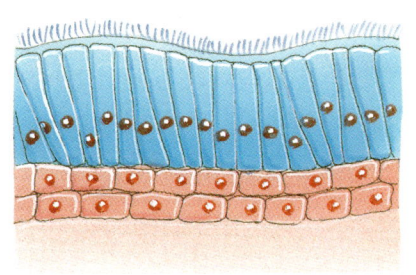

HEALTHY LUNG CELLS

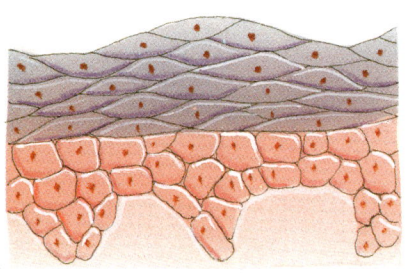

DAMAGED LUNG CELLS

Why do I yawn?

People often think that yawning is a sign of boredom, but this is not necessarily true. If you have not been breathing deeply for some time – usually when you are tired or have been sitting still – your reflexes force you to yawn and so take in more oxygen.

Why do some people snore?

People usually snore because they breathe through the mouth while asleep, often because their throat or nasal passages are blocked. The noise is caused by the vibration of a little projection of flesh at the back of the mouth known as the uvula as air moves over it.

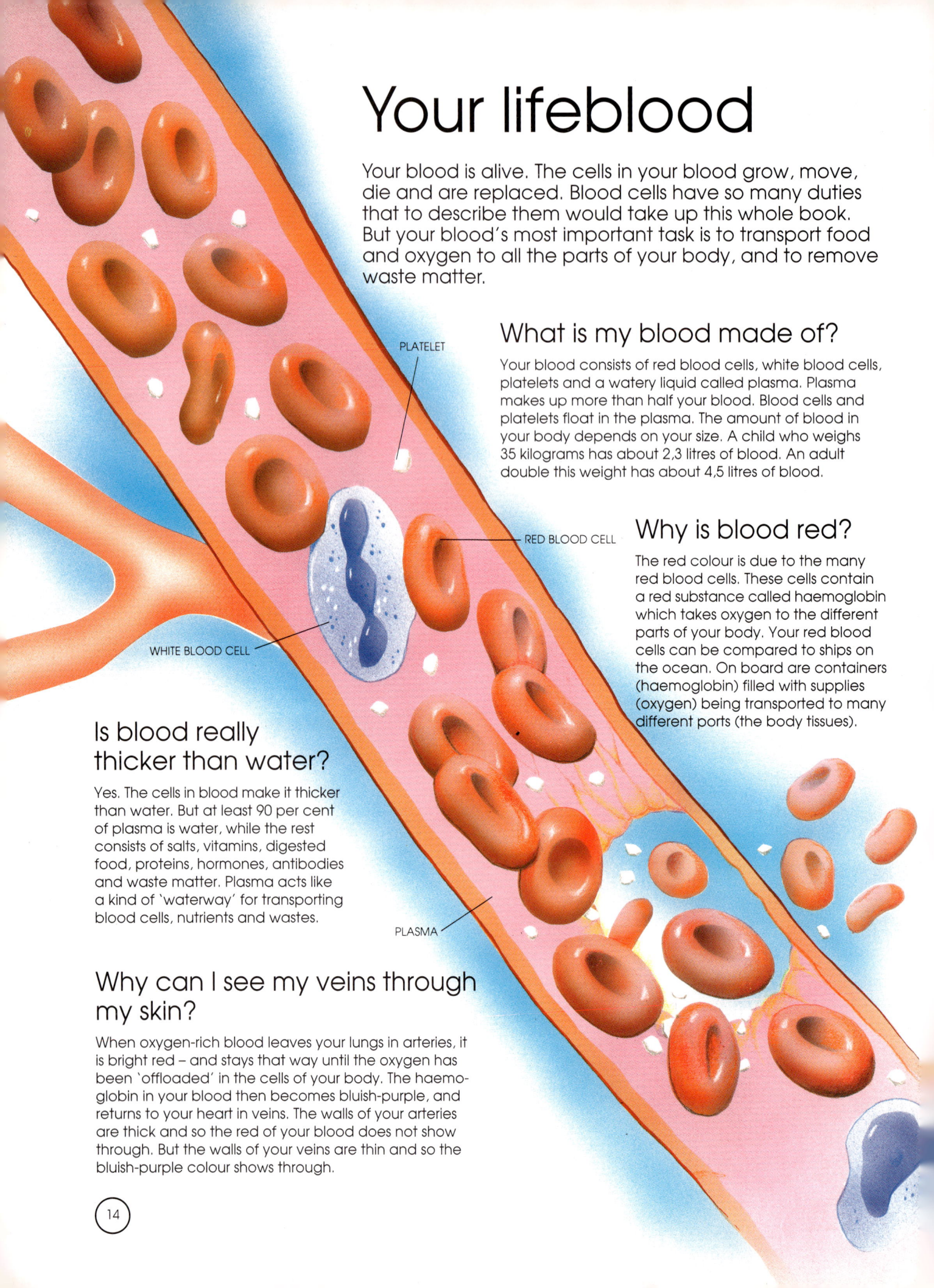

Your lifeblood

Your blood is alive. The cells in your blood grow, move, die and are replaced. Blood cells have so many duties that to describe them would take up this whole book. But your blood's most important task is to transport food and oxygen to all the parts of your body, and to remove waste matter.

PLATELET

What is my blood made of?

Your blood consists of red blood cells, white blood cells, platelets and a watery liquid called plasma. Plasma makes up more than half your blood. Blood cells and platelets float in the plasma. The amount of blood in your body depends on your size. A child who weighs 35 kilograms has about 2,3 litres of blood. An adult double this weight has about 4,5 litres of blood.

RED BLOOD CELL

Why is blood red?

The red colour is due to the many red blood cells. These cells contain a red substance called haemoglobin which takes oxygen to the different parts of your body. Your red blood cells can be compared to ships on the ocean. On board are containers (haemoglobin) filled with supplies (oxygen) being transported to many different ports (the body tissues).

WHITE BLOOD CELL

Is blood really thicker than water?

Yes. The cells in blood make it thicker than water. But at least 90 per cent of plasma is water, while the rest consists of salts, vitamins, digested food, proteins, hormones, antibodies and waste matter. Plasma acts like a kind of 'waterway' for transporting blood cells, nutrients and wastes.

PLASMA

Why can I see my veins through my skin?

When oxygen-rich blood leaves your lungs in arteries, it is bright red – and stays that way until the oxygen has been 'offloaded' in the cells of your body. The haemoglobin in your blood then becomes bluish-purple, and returns to your heart in veins. The walls of your arteries are thick and so the red of your blood does not show through. But the walls of your veins are thin and so the bluish-purple colour shows through.

Why don't I bleed to death when I cut my finger?

When you damage a small blood vessel, like those in your finger, the muscle in the vessel wall contracts and stops the blood from escaping from the cut. The platelets in your blood gather around the cut and stick to it and to themselves. As more platelets pile up they form a 'net' over the cut and a clot develops. The clot plugs the cut and stops more blood from being lost. A dried clot on the surface of your skin is called a scab.

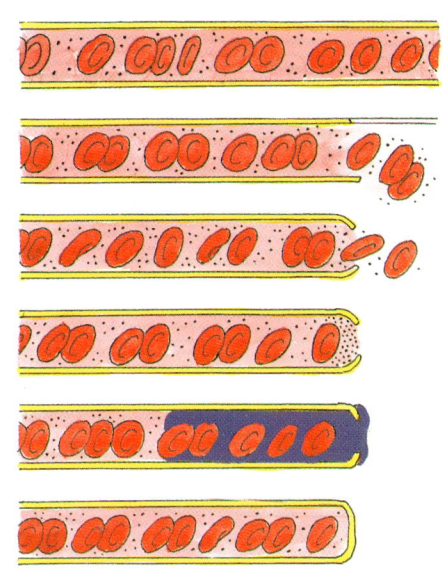

CLOTTING
Platelets stick together to form a scab

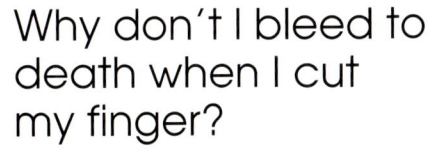

Bacteria

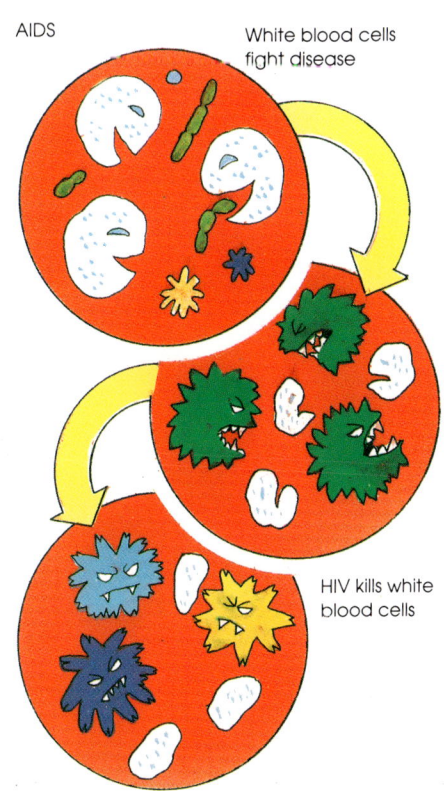

WHITE BLOOD CELLS
Cytoplasm swallows bacteria

AIDS

White blood cells fight disease

HIV kills white blood cells

Secondary diseases attack

Are there 'soldiers' in my blood?

Yes, your white blood cells act like soldiers to protect your body from disease. There are many different types of white blood cells. Some protect you by 'swallowing' bacteria or viruses and then killing them with substances called enzymes. Others make substances called antibodies which destroy the intruders. White blood cells are in fact not really white, but colourless.

What is AIDS?

AIDS stands for Acquired Immune Deficiency Syndrome. It is a disease caused when the Human Immuno Deficiency Virus (HIV) attacks the white blood cells and stops them from doing their job of fighting disease. AIDS often leads to death. You can get AIDS by having sex with an infected person, or if infected blood gets into your bloodstream. An infected pregnant mother can pass AIDS on to her unborn baby.

Did you know?

All fish, amphibians, reptiles, birds and mammals have red blood. Insects also have blood, but it does not contain haemoglobin and so is green or yellow, or sometimes even colourless.

How do nutrients and oxygen get from my blood to my cells?

Your arteries split up into smaller and smaller branches. The smallest of these are called capillaries. The walls of the capillaries are so thin that oxygen, nutrients and other substances pass from your blood vessels through them to your body cells. Carbon dioxide and other waste matter pass in the opposite direction. The capillaries then join up and form veins, which take the stale blood back to your heart. Your heart pumps your blood to your lungs for re-fuelling.

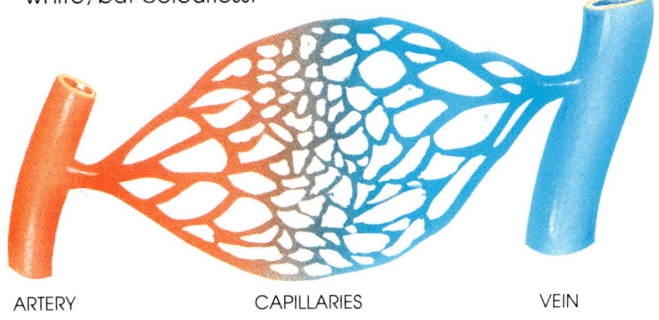

ARTERY   CAPILLARIES   VEIN

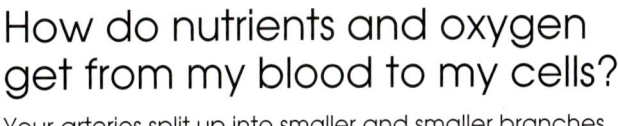

The headmaster

In order for a school to run smoothly, it has a headmaster or principal which controls all the activities in the school and makes important decisions. Your brain is your body's headmaster, controlling everything that happens in it and everything you do. It enables you to breathe, walk, talk, learn, remember, think, and feel happy and sad. Your brain makes you who you are.

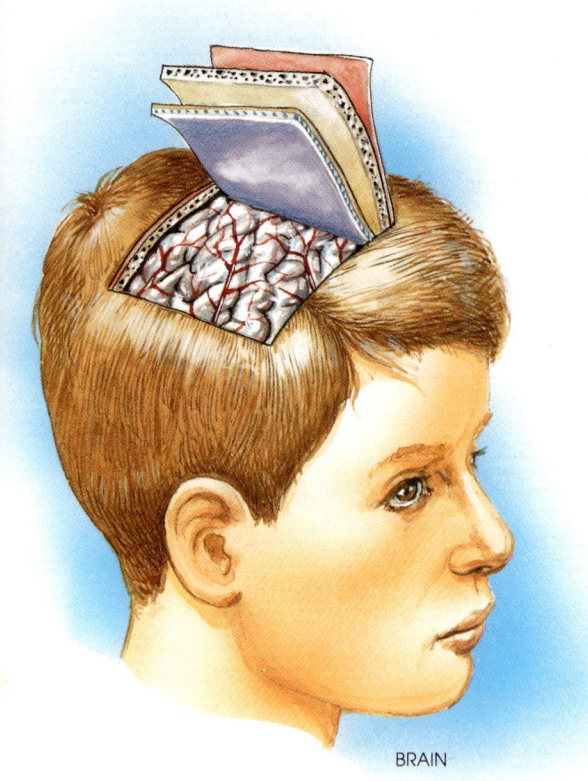

BRAIN

Is my brain in a box?

Yes, a box of bone. Because your brain is such an important organ, and because the cells of your brain do not regrow if they are damaged, your brain is very well protected from accidents. Just as a principal sits in an office at school, your brain has an 'office' in the upper part of your bony skull, sometimes called your 'brain box', or cranium. Although the skull is thin, its round shape makes it very strong indeed. For further protection and support, three membranes called meninges surround the brain.

Why do people sometimes call a brain a 'nut'?

Probably because it looks rather like a walnut without its shell. You have probably also heard people talking about their brains as their 'grey matter'. The outside of your brain is indeed grey – although the inside is white. The grey, outer part consists mostly of millions of nerve cell bodies (see page 18), perhaps even as many as 10 000 million! It is wrinkled to increase the area of its surface and so allow as many cells as possible to be packed in. Most of the white, inner part of your brain is made up of the nerve fibres from the nerve cell bodies in the grey layer.

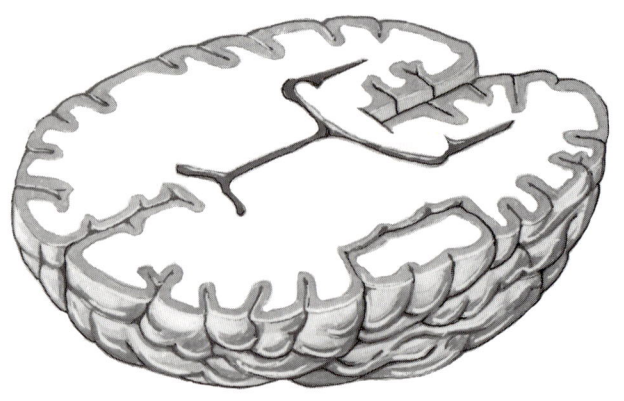

CROSS-SECTION
THROUGH THE BRAIN

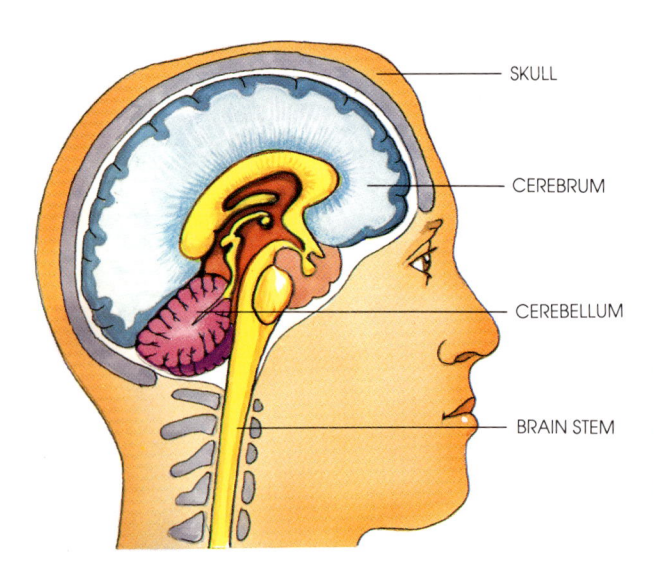

SKULL

CEREBRUM

CEREBELLUM

BRAIN STEM

Do I have only one brain?

Yes, but your brain is divided into three main parts, the cerebrum, the cerebellum and the brain stem. The cerebrum is the biggest part and fills the upper part of your head. It is divided in half by a deep groove. The cerebellum lies below the cerebrum, towards the back of your head. It is about the size of an orange. The brain stem connects the cerebrum, the cerebellum and the spinal cord. It is sausage-shaped and is about as thick as your thumb.

Does my brain give the orders?

Yes, but different parts of your brain give different orders. One of the most important tasks of the cerebrum is to receive information from your eyes, ears, nose, tongue and skin and to respond to this information. The cerebrum allows you to think, remember, talk, write and make decisions. Your feelings, moods and your personality are also controlled by the cerebrum. The cerebellum is responsible for your balance and co-ordination. Together with the spinal cord your brain stem controls bodily functions such as breathing and heart beat. It also allows you to go to sleep and wake up again. Scientists think that memories are not stored in any one part of the brain, but all over.

Which side of my brain do I use to do maths?

If you are right-handed, you most probably use the left side of your brain to do logical things (things that need working out), such as maths, science experiments and playing chess. The right side of your brain controls your artistic and musical abilities. The opposite happens if you are left-handed. But did you know that the right side of your body is linked to the left side of your brain? The nerve fibres in the nerves connecting your brain and spinal cord cross over before going into your cerebrum.

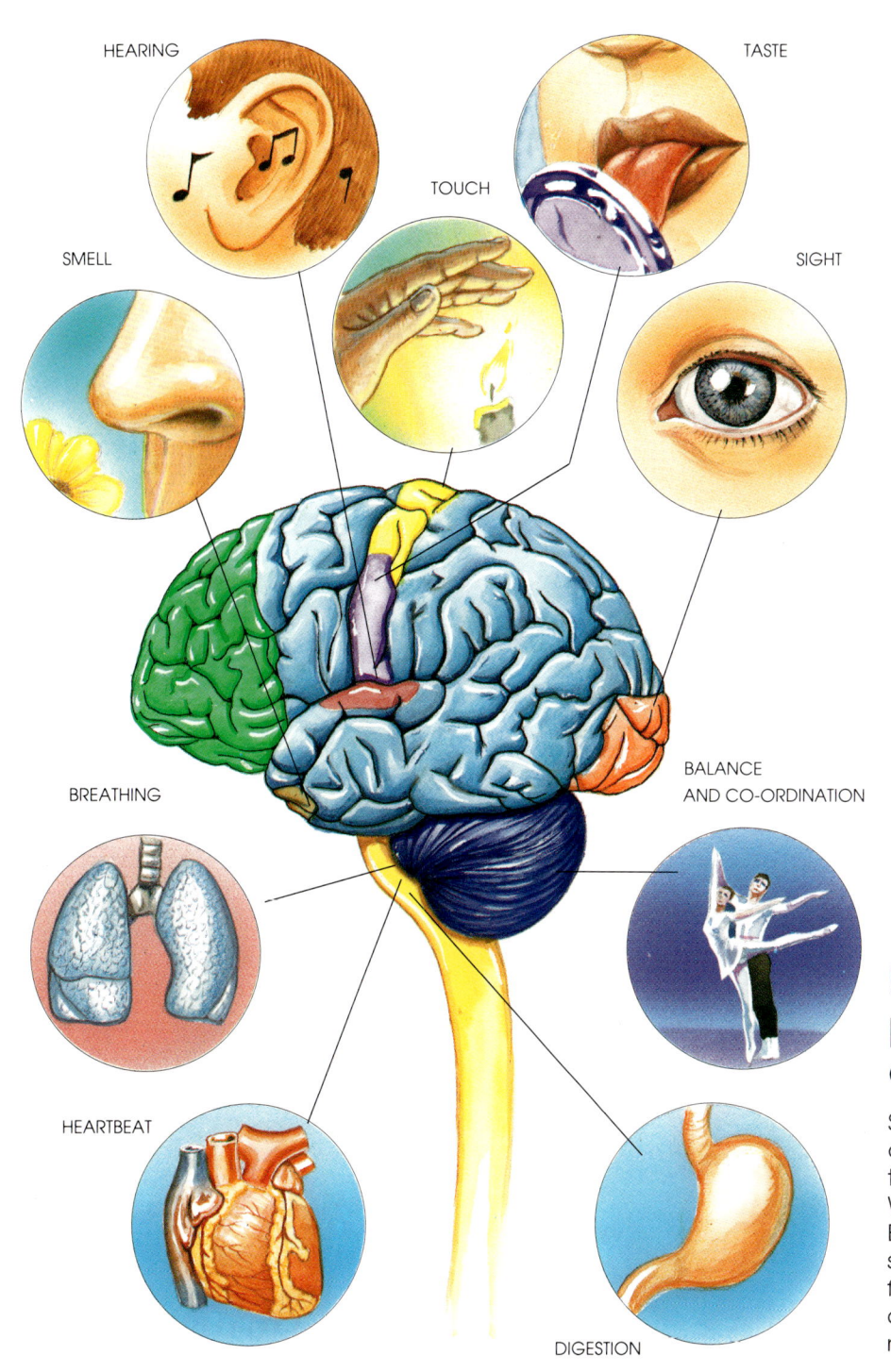

HEARING · TASTE · TOUCH · SMELL · SIGHT · BREATHING · BALANCE AND CO-ORDINATION · HEARTBEAT · DIGESTION

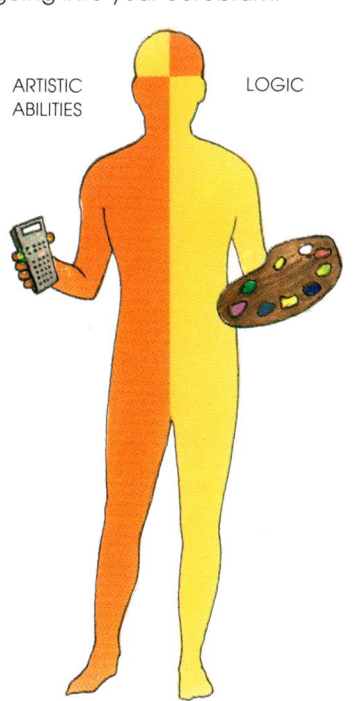

ARTISTIC ABILITIES · LOGIC

Does a 'brainy' person's brain look any different?

Scientists have been unable to find anything physically different about the brain of a very clever person. When the great physicist Albert Einstein died in 1955, scientists studied his brain in the hope of finding the reason for his remarkable intelligence. His brain looked no different from anyone else's.

Cell body

Getting the message across

Your spinal cord, which runs from your brain about two-thirds of the way down your backbone, works very closely with your brain. Together, they control everything you do.

Does my brain reach down my back?

Almost. Your spinal cord is actually an extension of your brain. It is a long, thick bundle of nerve fibres connecting your brain to the rest of your body. It is just thicker than a pencil, and has a small hole running down its centre. Just as your brain is safely enclosed in your skull, your spinal cord is surrounded by a set of bones called vertebrae. The vertebrae make up your spinal column. Between each vertebra is a narrow gap through which nerves pass from your spinal cord to your body.

Dendrite

Axon

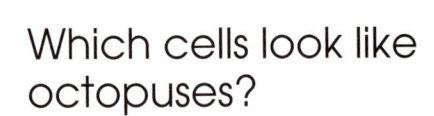

NERVE CELL

Which cells look like octopuses?

Your nerve cells, or neurons. Each consists of a ball-shaped cell body with a nucleus, and lots of branching nerve fibres called dendrites sticking out from the sides, making the cell look a bit like an octopus. Each nerve cell has an additional arm or nerve fibre called an axon. The axon is sometimes branched and can be very long – those running from your spine to your toes can be more than a metre long!

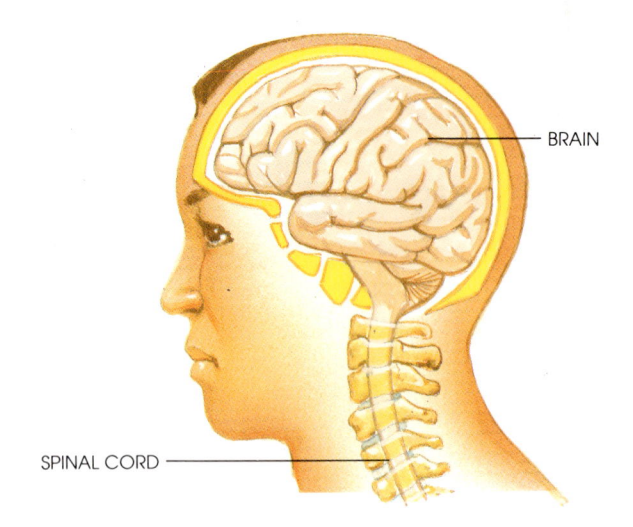

BRAIN

SPINAL CORD

How many nerve cells are there in my body?

Between 10 000 million and 100 000 million! Most are in your brain. Although you have so many nerve cells, your nerves have only two main types of nerve fibres: sensory nerve fibres, which carry messages from your sense organs (like your eyes) to your brain and spinal cord; and motor nerve fibres, which carry messages from your brain and spinal cord to your muscles and other parts of your body. Most nerves contain both types of fibres.

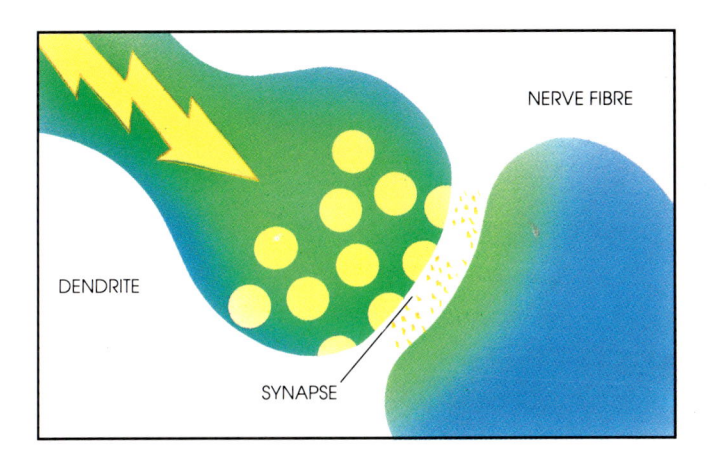

NERVE FIBRE

DENDRITE

SYNAPSE

Is there electricity running through my body?

Yes. Messages are passed along the nerve fibres in the form of very weak electrical signals. If you prick a finger, nerve endings in your skin (see page 20) pick up the information and send it along nerve fibres to your spinal cord. Surprisingly, no two nerve fibres are ever joined. They are separated from one another by a tiny gap called a synapse. Electrical signals 'jump' across this gap with the help of chemicals.

How do my nerves help me when I'm in danger?

If you see a bull charging towards you, electrical signals flash from your eyes to your brain. The nerve cells in your brain receive this information, examine it, and decide what should be done about it. A message saying 'charging bull' means danger. So your brain then immediately sends messages saying 'run' to your muscles and other parts of your body. The muscles in your legs get the message, and immediately put your legs into action!

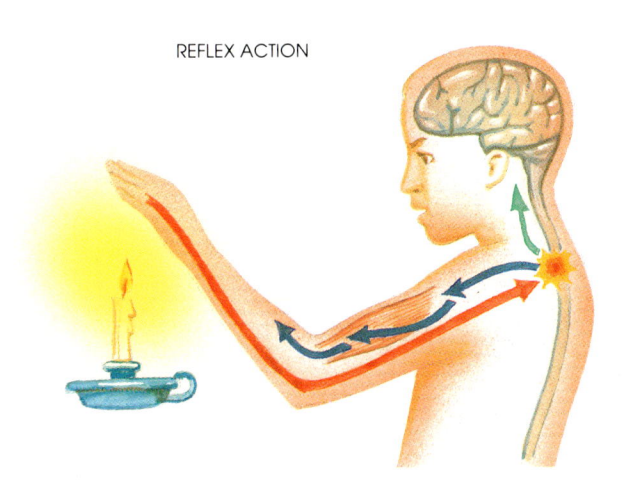

REFLEX ACTION

Why do I pull my finger away so quickly when I burn it?

Sometimes your body needs to react very quickly, without waiting for a message from your brain. If you were to accidentally burn your finger on a hot-plate, tiny sense organs in your skin (see page 20) would immediately send a message saying 'pain' to your spinal cord. Your spinal cord would then send signals instructing your arm muscles to 'pull', and so jerk your finger away from the heat. Doing something without thinking about it is known as reflex action.

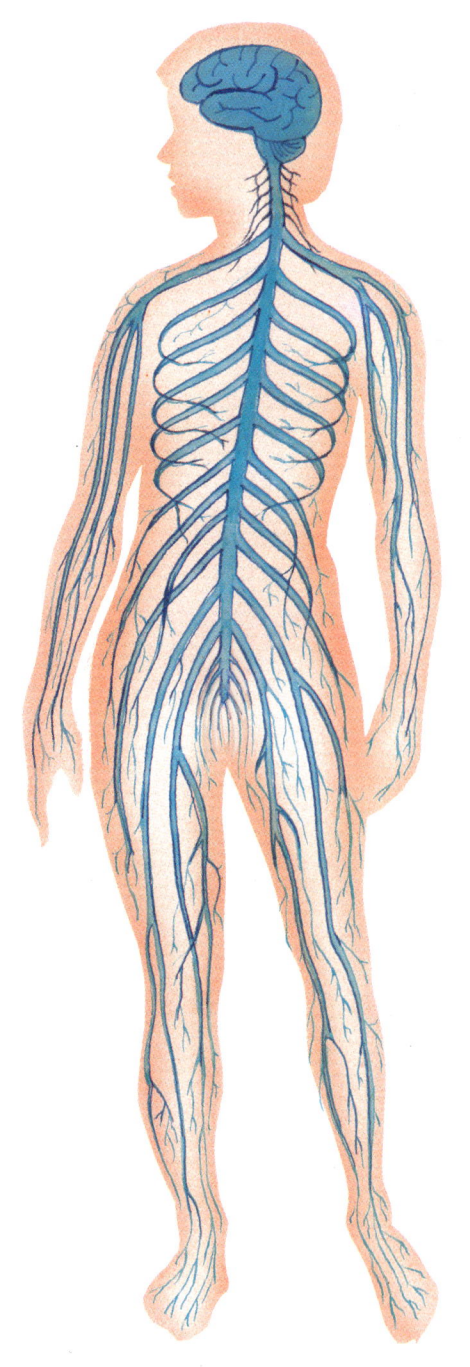

HUMAN NERVOUS SYSTEM

Under cover

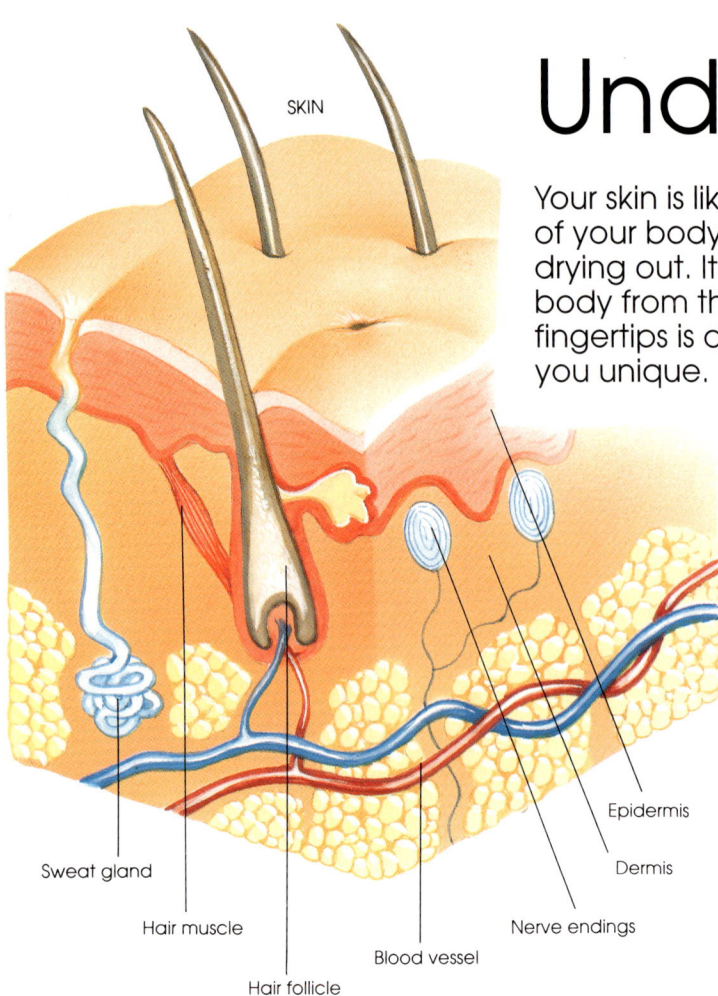

SKIN

Your skin is like close-fitting clothing, following every curve of your body. It is waterproof and stops your body from drying out. It keeps harmful germs out. It protects your body from the sun. And because the pattern on your fingertips is different from anyone else's, your skin makes you unique.

Sweat gland

Hair muscle

Hair follicle

Blood vessel

Nerve endings

Epidermis

Dermis

Am I dead on the outside?

Yes. Your skin has two layers. The top layer of your skin, the epidermis, has many dead cells on its surface – although the cells at the bottom of this layer are alive and active. These cells continually split to make more new cells, which are then pushed to the surface of your skin where they die. The cells of the epidermis contain a substance called keratin, which makes your skin waterproof and germproof. The epidermis protects the sensitive lower layer of your skin.

If I prick a finger, where do I feel the pain?

In the lower layer of your skin, or dermis. This layer contains many different structures, each with a different job. Among these are nerve endings which feel pain, heat, cold and pressure. Special little organs measure the amount of pain, heat, cold and pressure. Also in the dermis are special glands that produce oil to keep your skin soft and waterproof, blood vessels that bring food and oxygen to your skin, sweat glands, and hair roots.

Why don't my nails hurt when I cut them?

Your nails are made of dead keratin cells and have no feeling. A nail consists of a root, covered by skin called the cuticle, and a nail plate, which is the part you can see. At the bottom of the nail plate you can sometimes see a small white crescent called a lunula, meaning 'little moon'. Your nails shield the tips of your fingers and toes, and help you do 'fiddly' things like thread a needle.

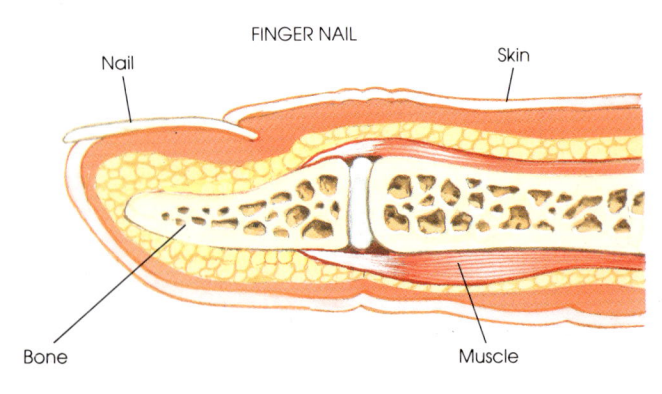

FINGER NAIL

Nail

Skin

Bone

Muscle

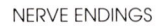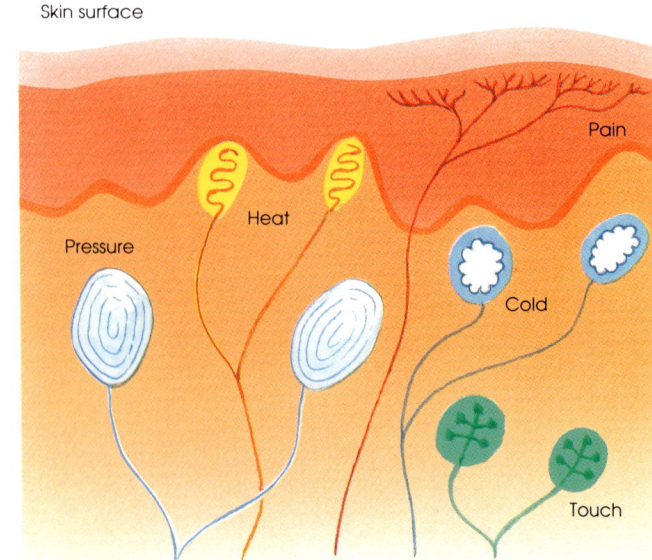

NERVE ENDINGS

Skin surface

Pain

Heat

Pressure

Cold

Touch

Why do I get goose bumps?

Goose bumps help keep your body warm. Every hair in your skin has a tiny muscle attached to it. When you get cold, these muscles contract and pull the hairs upright. At the same time, the muscles push the skin around the hairs up, forming goose bumps. This traps air between the hairs and helps keep you warm. Your hair has many other functions. The hairs on your head protect you from the harmful rays of the sun and cushion your head when you bump it. The hairs in your nose trap and clear away dust particles. Your eyebrows soak up sweat from your forehead to protect your eyes.

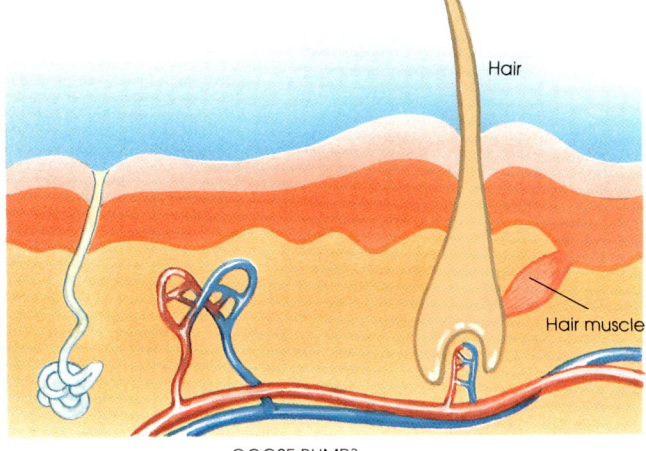

GOOSE BUMPS

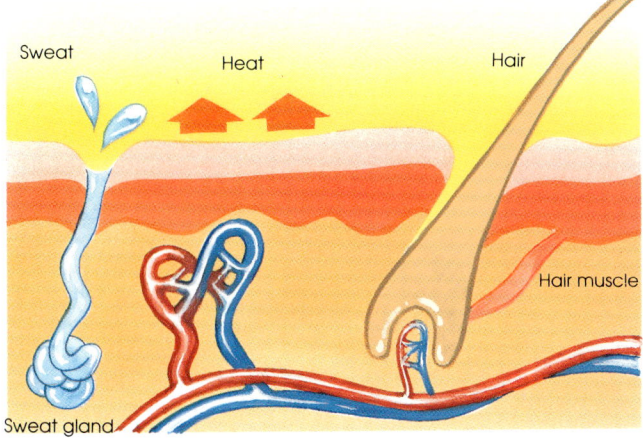

SWEATING

How does my skin cool my body down?

When your body gets hot, long, curly sweat glands in the skin produce sweat which leaves your body through pores on your skin. As the sweat evaporates, it draws heat from your body, so cooling you down. The blood vessels in your skin also help keep you cool. When you are hot, the vessels widen and bring more blood to the surface of your body, where it can lose heat to the air outside and then cool down. When you are cold, the blood vessels get narrower so that you lose less heat.

What gives skin its colour?

Much of the colour is due to a substance called melanin, made by cells at the bottom of the epidermis. Melanin protects the deeper parts of the skin from the dangerous rays of the sun, and so people from hot, sunny parts of the world need more of it than people from cooler places. So the cells of dark-skinned people make more melanin than those of fair-skinned people. The pink colour in skin comes from the blood in the tiny vessels in your skin.

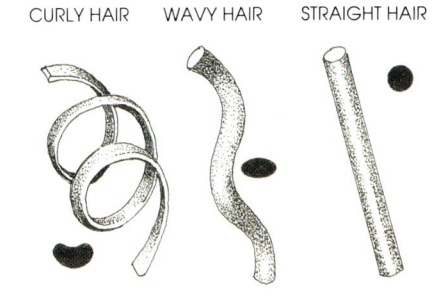

CURLY HAIR   WAVY HAIR   STRAIGHT HAIR

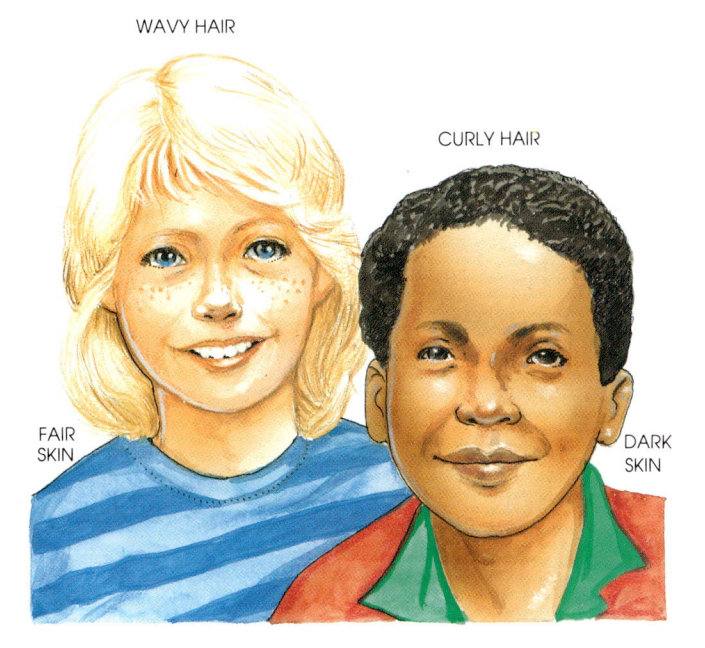

WAVY HAIR

CURLY HAIR

FAIR SKIN

DARK SKIN

What makes hair straight or curly?

Your hair follicles, deep pits in your skin from which your hair grows, give hair its shape. If you were to cut a hair and looked at it under a microscope, the shape of the cut end would tell you about the rest of the hair. If the cut end were round, your hair would be straight; if oval, your hair would be wavy; and if bean-shaped, your hair would be very curly.

Why do I peel?

When you stay in the sun for a long time, your skin makes more melanin to help shade your body and so it goes darker. Too much sun destroys the cells of the epidermis and they are replaced by new cells. The damaged cells are then pushed to the surface of your skin where they peel off. The ultraviolet rays of the sun can be dangerous, so always use a barrier cream when you are in the sun.

Windows on the world

Your eyes are sense organs, because they tell you what is going on around you. They allow you to see spectacular sunsets, watch television, play sport, spot danger and so run from it – and do many other things. Eyes are one of your most valuable possessions.

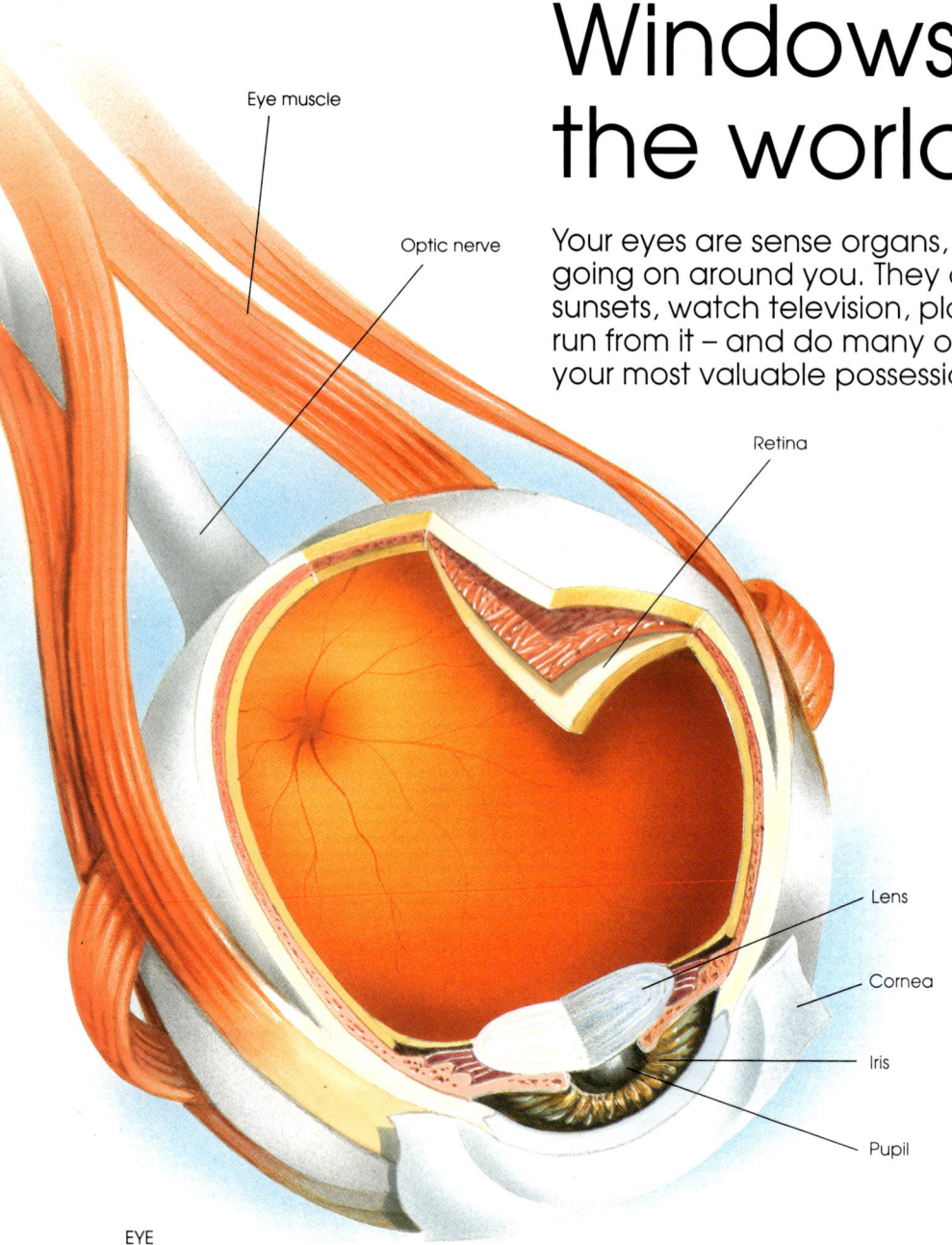

Eye muscle

Optic nerve

Retina

Lens

Cornea

Iris

Pupil

EYE

Could my eyes pop out of my head?

No. Your eyes are safely encased in bony sockets in the front of your skull. The bone behind the eyebrows sticks out like a car bumper to protect the eyes from knocks, and the eyes rest on fatty tissue which cushions them against shock. Eyebrows and eyelashes stop dust and sweat getting into the eyes. But eyebrows also show your feelings by giving expression to your face.

Why are my eyes round?

So that they can move freely in the sockets of your skull. They are filled with a jelly-like substance which keeps their shape, just as air gives a balloon its shape. Each eye has a 'window' called a cornea. Behind it is a coloured ring, the iris, with a hole in the middle, the pupil. Six muscles control the eyeball's movement.

Why are eyes different colours?

The colour of your eyes depends on the amount of melanin (see page 21) in your irises. The more melanin you have, the darker your eyes are. So people with dark brown or black eyes have lots of melanin, people with light brown eyes less. Blue eyes are not caused by blue melanin, but rather because the iris contains very little melanin.

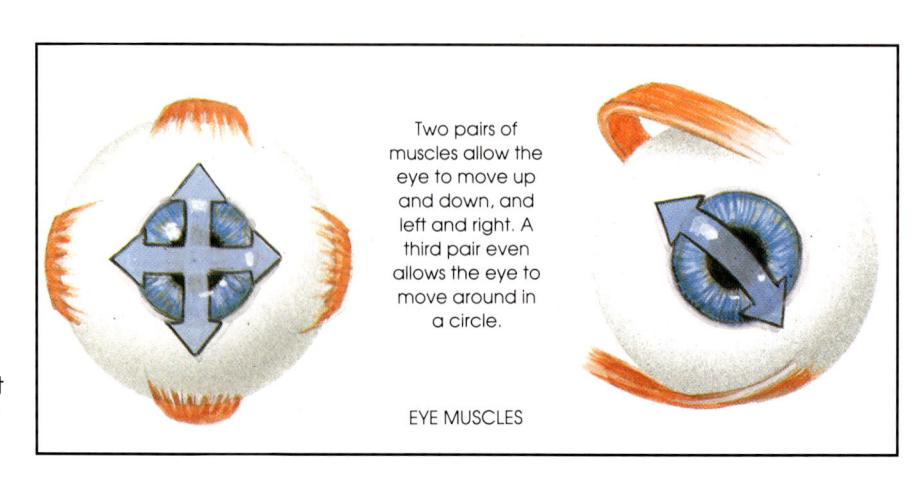

Two pairs of muscles allow the eye to move up and down, and left and right. A third pair even allows the eye to move around in a circle.

EYE MUSCLES

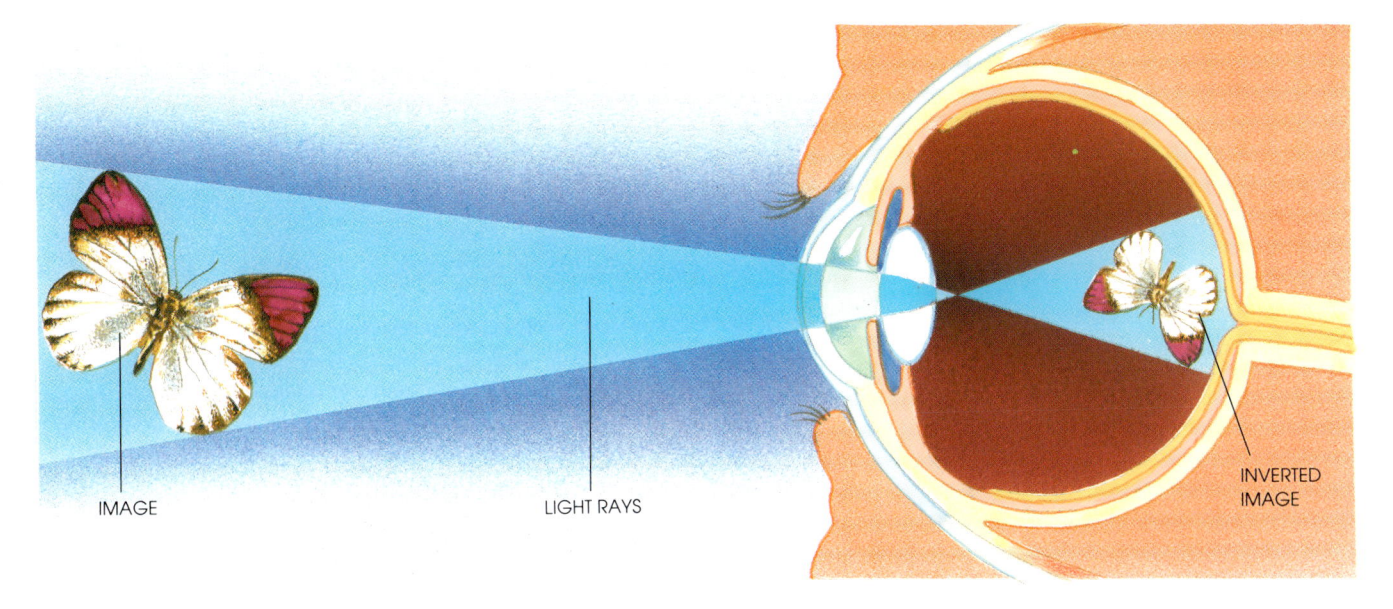

IMAGE

LIGHT RAYS

INVERTED IMAGE

Is my eye like a camera?

Yes, your eye takes pictures rather like a camera does. When you look at a butterfly, for example, light rays from the butterfly pass through your cornea and pupil, and are focused by a see-through lens. The amount of light that comes in is controlled by the iris, which opens and closes like a camera shutter. The lens turns the light rays upside down and focuses them on the retina at the back of your eye, just as a camera lens focuses light rays onto film. The eye's optic nerve takes the upside down picture from the retina to the brain. Your brain turns the picture the right way up again – and tells you that you are seeing a butterfly.

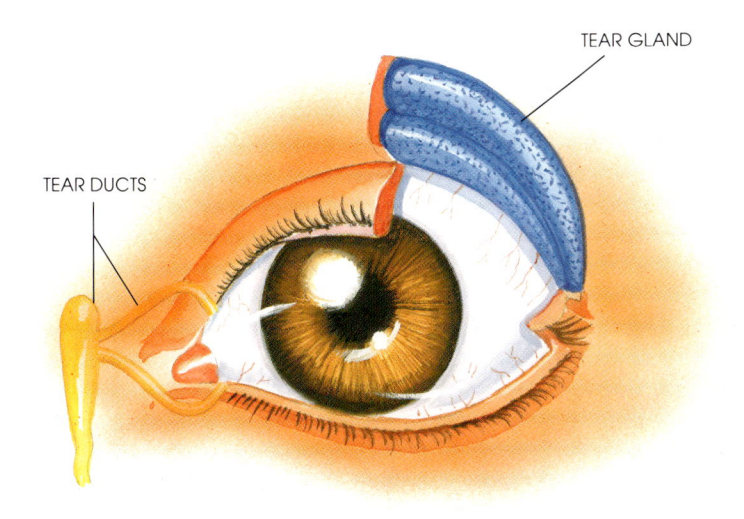

TEAR GLAND

TEAR DUCTS

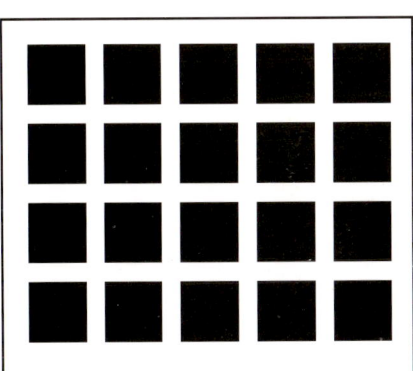

Did you know?

Your eyes really do play tricks on you. When you look at certain patterns, your brain is slightly confused and gives you wrong information based on what it expects to see. Take a look at the series of black blocks in the picture above. You should see grey spots jumping about at the intersections of the blocks. Seeing something that is not really there – like the grey spots – is known as an optical illusion.

Where do my tears come from?

Your tears come from a tiny tear gland on the top, outer edge of each eye. They flow over the eyes and then pass into two tiny canals, the tear ducts, in the inner corner of each eye. A tube then carries the tears into your nose. When you cry or laugh heartily, or when you stand near chopped onion, your glands make more fluid than your ducts can take in – and the tears roll down your cheeks and sometimes even from your nose!

Are there 'shutters' on my eyes?

If your eyes are like windows, then your eyelids are like shutters which close to protect your eyes. When you blink, your eyelids spread tear fluid over your eyes, washing away germs and stopping your corneas from drying out. You also blink if an object suddenly moves close to your eyes. Your eyelids, which contain a tough sheet of cartilage (see page 7), also close to guard your eyeballs while you sleep.

On the air

We live in a completely silent world! Sound is actually a series of vibrations picked up by your ears and interpreted as noise by your brain. But your ears do not work on their own. They are connected by tubes to your nose. Together with your throat, your ear and nose allow you to hear, smell, speak, swallow, take in air and keep your balance.

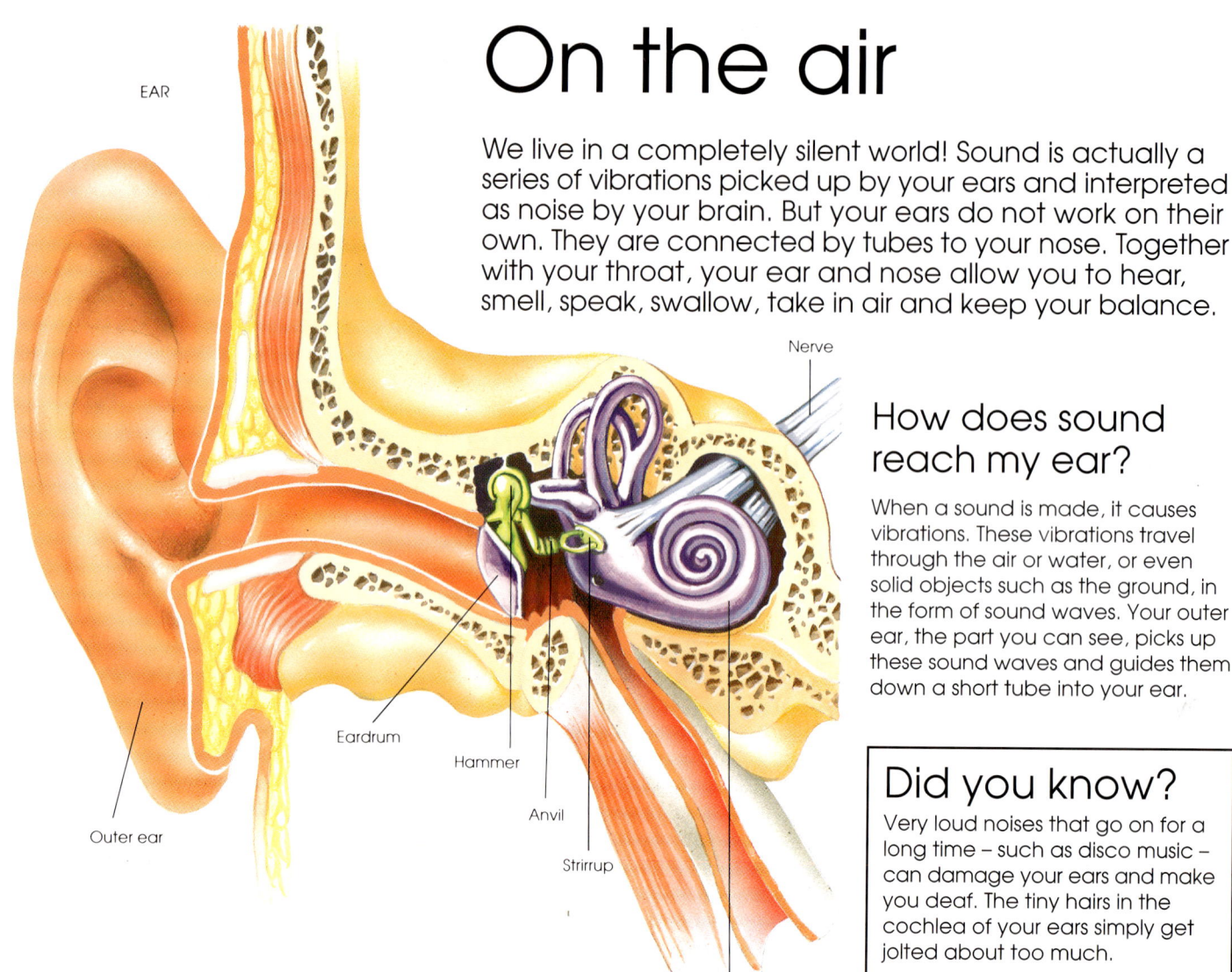

EAR

Outer ear

Eardrum

Hammer

Anvil

Strirrup

Nerve

Cochlea

How does sound reach my ear?

When a sound is made, it causes vibrations. These vibrations travel through the air or water, or even solid objects such as the ground, in the form of sound waves. Your outer ear, the part you can see, picks up these sound waves and guides them down a short tube into your ear.

Did you know?

Very loud noises that go on for a long time – such as disco music – can damage your ears and make you deaf. The tiny hairs in the cochlea of your ears simply get jolted about too much.

Is my eardrum really like a drum?

Almost. Your eardrum is a tiny piece of skin stretched across the inside of your ear, just as the membrane of a drum is stretched across a hollow cylinder. Sound waves coming into your ear first hit your eardrum, causing it to vibrate. The vibrations pass to your middle ear, a small chamber with three tiny bones called the hammer, anvil and stirrup, named for their shapes. Although these bones are the tiniest in your body, they make the sounds even louder, and then send the vibrations to another chamber, the inner ear.

Are there snails in my ears?

No, of course not. But inside each of your two inner ears is a snail-shaped cochlea. This tube is filled with a liquid and lined with thousands of tiny hairs connected to nerve cells. These cells turn the sound vibrations into electric signals (see page 19), which travel to your brain where they are interpreted as sound.

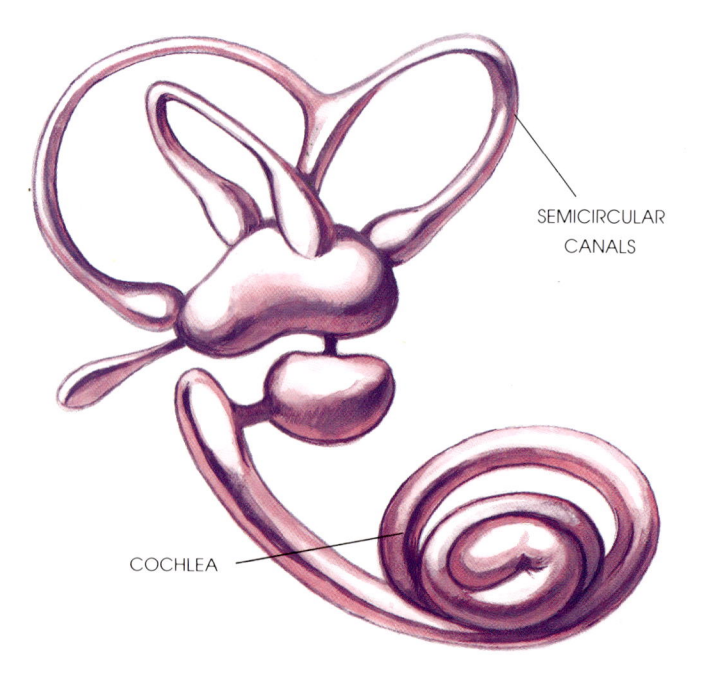

SEMICIRCULAR CANALS

COCHLEA

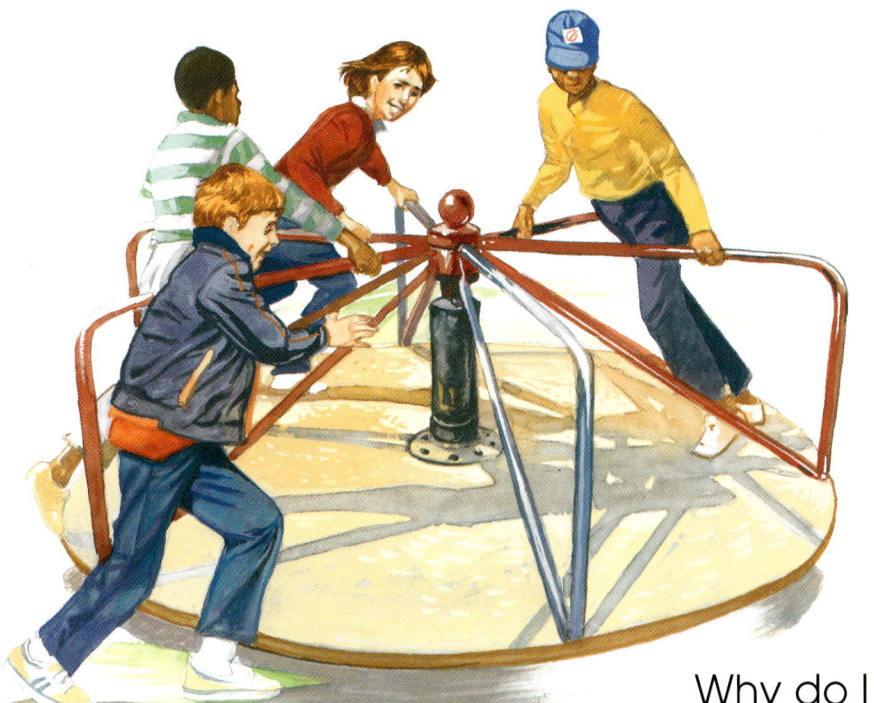

Why do I get dizzy when I spin around?

Your ears not only let you hear, but give you a sense of balance. Inside your inner ear, above the cochlea, are three looped semicircular canals. These canals contain liquid and are lined with little hairs connected to nerve endings. When you move your head, the liquid in the loops swirls about and bends the hairs, telling your brain in which direction you are moving. If you spin round and round and suddenly stop, the liquid goes on swirling, even though you are no longer moving. Your brain cannot tell what's going on, and you feel dizzy.

Why do I have two ears?

So that you can tell from which direction a sound is coming. If a dog standing on your right barks at you, the sound waves reach your right ear a fraction of a second before they reach your left ear. Your brain detects the time difference and tells you that the sound is coming from your right.

How does the air help me to smell?

It carries smells to your nose and up your nostrils! Although one of the most important jobs of your nose is to warm and filter the air before it goes into your lungs, a small part is used to smell. Inside the top of your nose are two patches made up of about 10 million receptor cells, which are covered by a layer of sticky mucus and are connected to nerve fibres leading to your brain. Each cell has a few fine hairs sticking out into the mucus. It is these hairs which detect smells carried through the air.

What is my Adam's apple?

Your voice box, or larynx, which is a tube-shaped structure made mostly of cartilage. It works with your tongue and lips so you can speak. Your Adam's apple lies at the top of your windpipe. Stretched across the inside of your voice box are two flaps known as your vocal cords. When you breathe, your cords are relaxed and air passes freely through the gap between them. When you speak, your cords move closer together. Air is forced through the narrow gap, causing the cords to vibrate and produce sounds. Your tongue and lips shape the sounds into words.

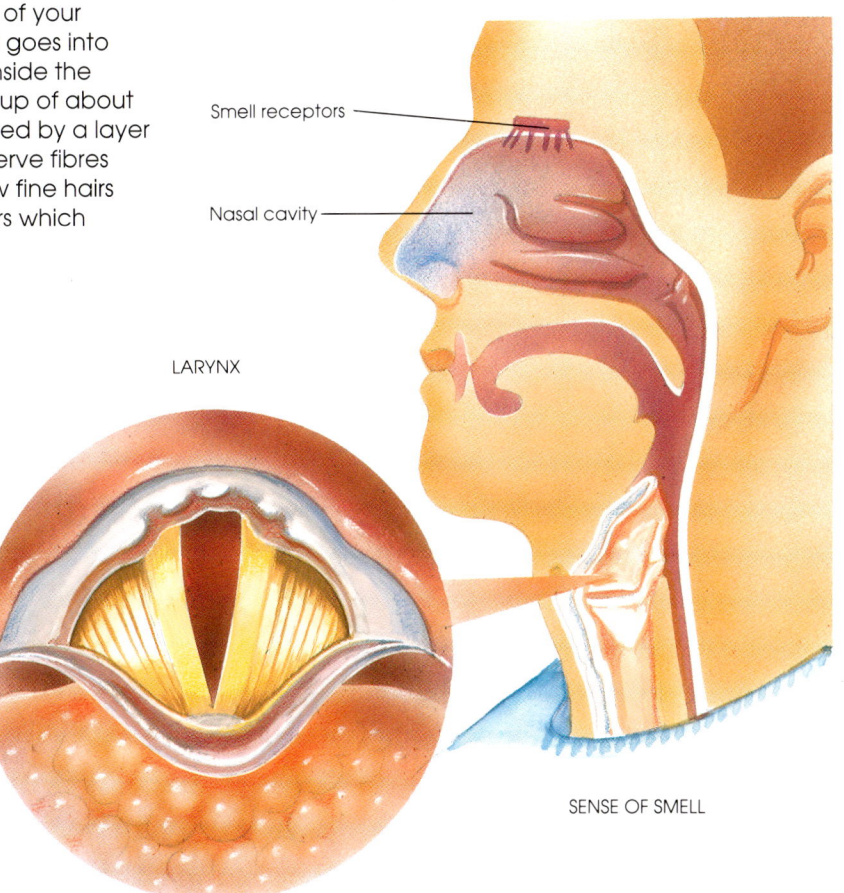

Smell receptors

Nasal cavity

LARYNX

SENSE OF SMELL

A bite to eat

Food is essential for life. But it is useless to your body unless it is crushed and chopped into its smallest chemical parts. This process is known as digestion, and takes place in a long tube called the gut, or alimentary canal, which stretches from your mouth to your anus.

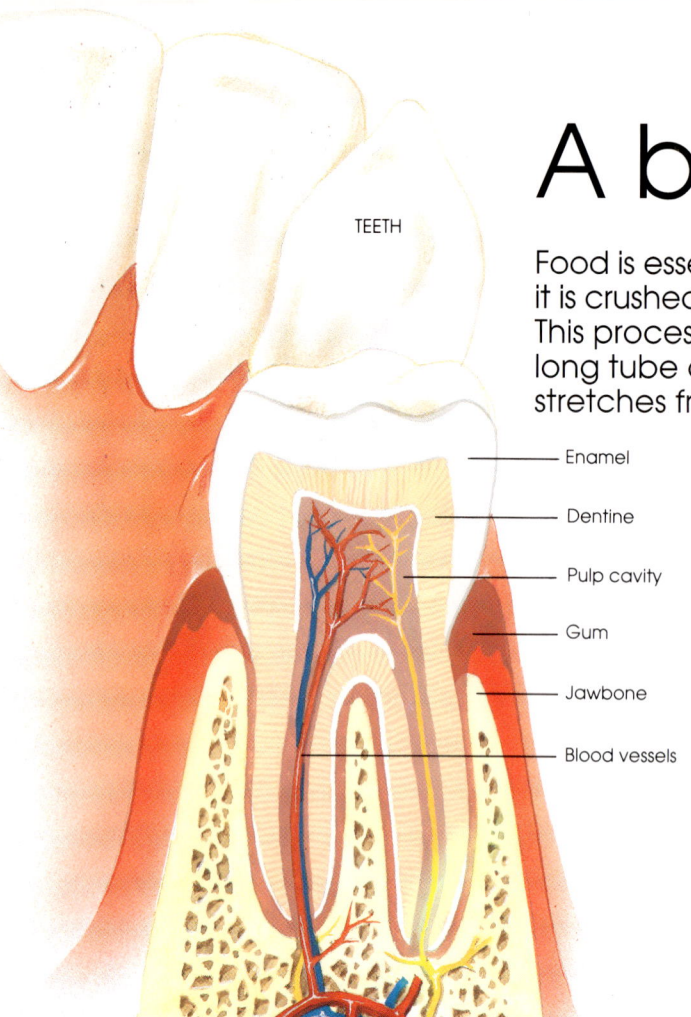

TEETH

— Enamel

— Dentine

— Pulp cavity

— Gum

— Jawbone

— Blood vessels

Where does digestion begin?

In the mouth. Your teeth, with the help of your tongue, cut and crush food and break it down. Three pairs of glands in your mouth give off a liquid called saliva, which moistens your food and helps it stick together so that it is easier to swallow. Saliva contains substances called enzymes which begin to break down certain foods. Saliva also helps kill bacteria, and helps keep your mouth clean by washing away bits of food.

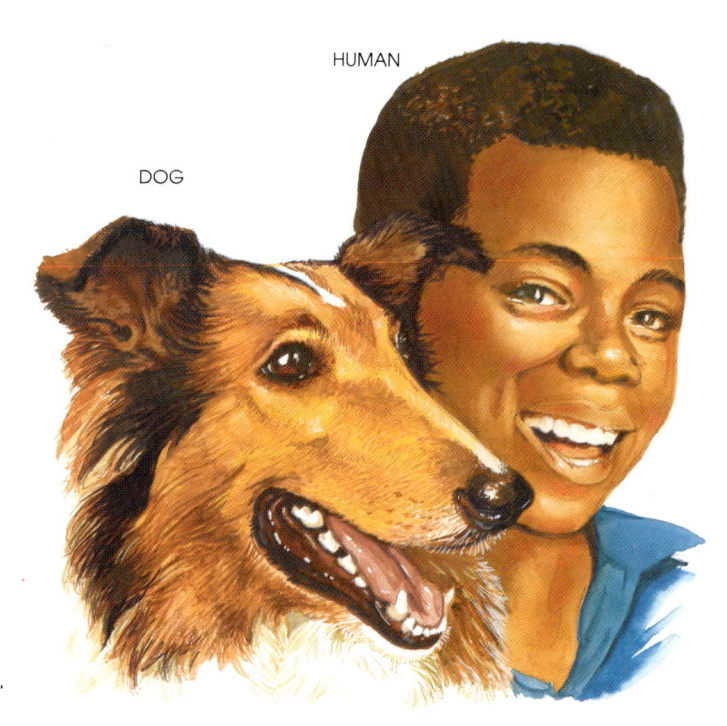

HUMAN

DOG

Why are my teeth different from a cat or dog's teeth?

Because you eat different food. Meat-eating animals have long, piercing fangs to grip and tear raw flesh. People eat many different foods, and have four kinds of teeth to cut and crush these foods into smaller bits. Your eight front teeth (in your upper and lower jaws) are called incisors. They bite off bits of food. Your next four teeth (on either side of your incisors) are called canines. They tear tough foods. Next are premolars and molars. They are flattish and crush and grind food.

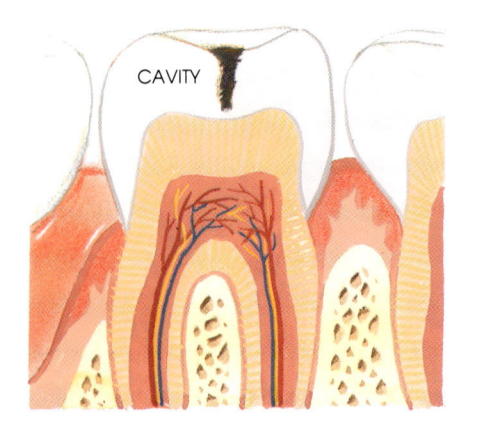

CAVITY

Why do I get toothache?

The inside of your teeth – an area called the pulp – contains many nerves and blood vessels, and is covered by a hard substance called dentine. The part of your tooth which sticks out above the gum is surrounded by another hard, protective layer called enamel. Bits of food in your mouth give off acid and if your teeth are not cleaned regularly, the acid slowly destroys the enamel and dentine. As the damage spreads into the pulp, your teeth begin to ache because the sensitive nerves are exposed. The part of your teeth set into your gums is known as the root. In your first year, the first of about 20 milk teeth begin to appear, and from about the age of six, they are replaced by 32 permanent teeth.

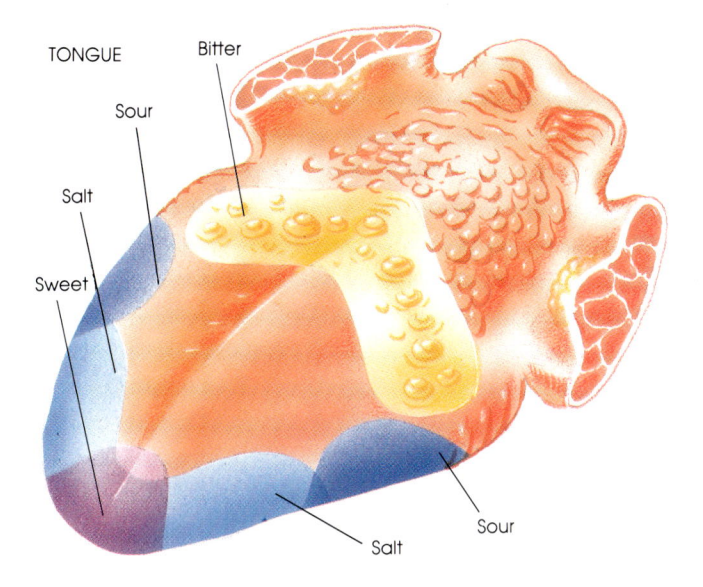

TONGUE
Bitter
Sour
Salt
Sweet
Sour
Salt

Are the bumps on my tongue my taste buds?

Not quite. The little bumps on the surface of your tongue are tiny growths called papillae. They make your tongue rough to help break down food. But at the bottom of some of the papillae is a group of sense cells connected to a nerve. These cells form your taste buds, which detect the flavour of the food in your mouth. Different areas of your tongue pick out four different flavours: sweet, sour, bitter and salty. Your tongue also does many other useful things. It helps you to speak. It moves food about while you chew so that your teeth can get to it and so that saliva can be mixed into it. It helps you swallow by pushing food to the back of your mouth, and warns you when foods are too hot or bad.

What would happen if I ate upside down?

Food would pass into your oesophagus – a tube which leads from your mouth to your stomach – even if you were upside down! The muscles in the walls of the oesophagus automatically contract and narrow the tube just behind the food, forcing the food on towards the stomach. This squeezing action is known as peristalsis. When you swallow, a small flap of tissue called the epiglottis closes off the entrance to your windpipe. At the same time, another flap of tissue closes off the tube leading to your nose. This prevents food from slipping into your lungs and nose.

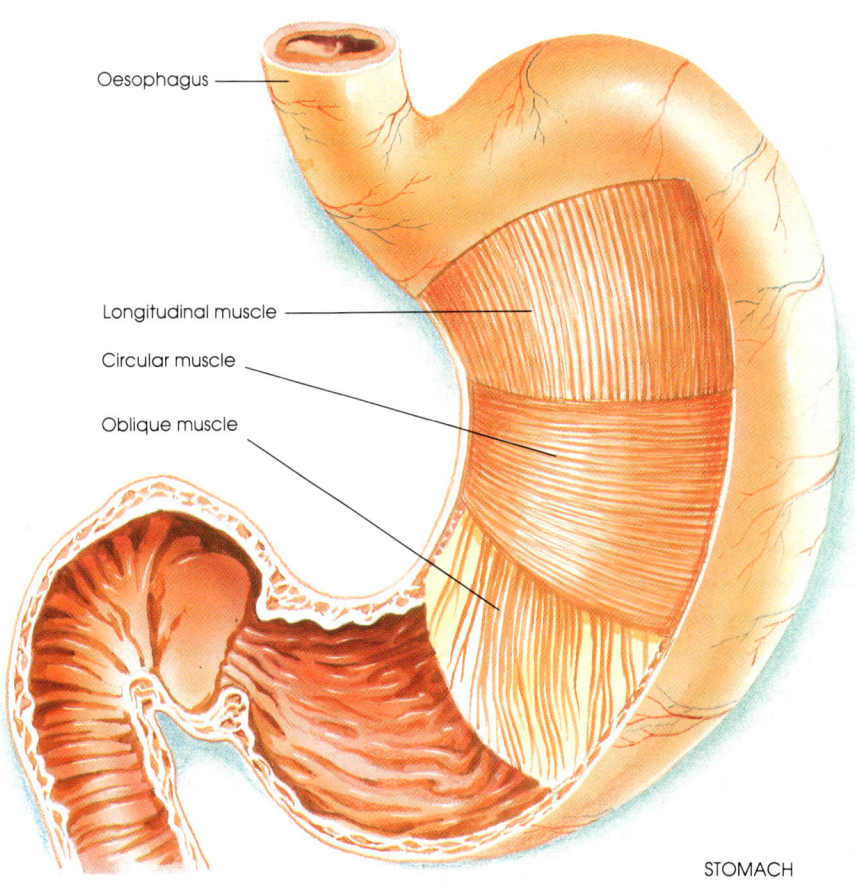

Oesophagus
Longitudinal muscle
Circular muscle
Oblique muscle
STOMACH

PERISTALSIS

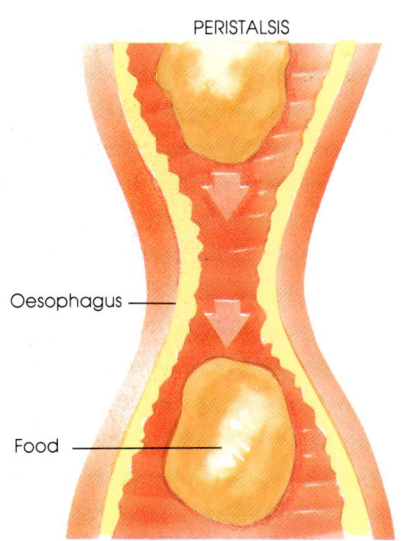

Oesophagus
Food

Why does my stomach rumble?

Your stomach and intestines are always making noises, but you do not always hear them. Most of the thick, strong walls of the stomach consist of muscles which contract and relax to stir, squeeze and churn the food about. The rumbles you hear when you are hungry are caused by the contracting and relaxing of the muscles, and are amplified by the 'emptiness' of your stomach and intestines. The rumbles seem to stop after you have eaten, and after about two hours the food leaves your stomach and passes to your small intestine.

Food for life

Once your food has been broken down into its smallest parts, the nutrients are able to pass through the walls of your intestines into your blood, which carries them to different parts of your body. Food gives your body energy to build new cells, repair old ones and fight disease. The undigested or unwanted parts of your food then pass out of your body.

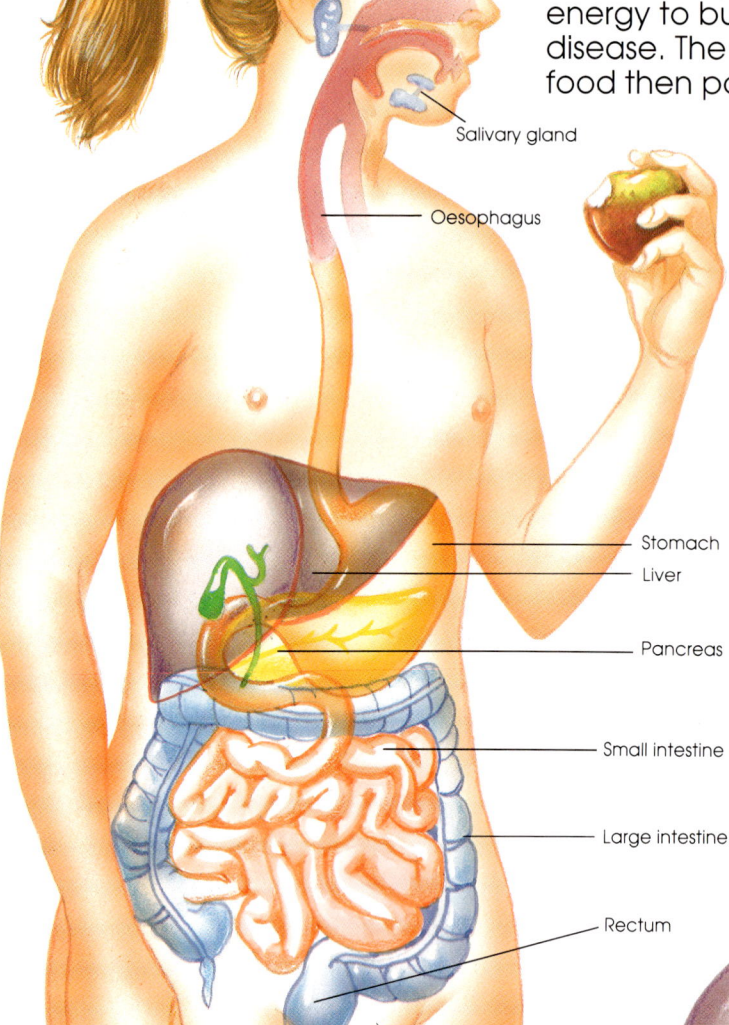

Salivary gland

Oesophagus

Stomach
Liver
Pancreas
Small intestine
Large intestine
Rectum

DIGESTIVE SYSTEM

Why is my liver red?

Because it has a very large blood supply. In fact, about a quarter of all your blood flows through this organ. Your liver has many different jobs. The liver stores important substances like vitamins and glucose. It removes or destroys poisonous substances in your blood. And it helps digestion by making a bitter, green liquid called bile which breaks down fat. Bile is stored in a small organ under your liver called the gall bladder, and passes through a tube called the bile duct to the small intestine when it is needed.

What is a pancreas?

Your pancreas is a leaf-shaped gland lying just below your stomach, and is connected to your small intestine by a tube called the pancreatic duct. It produces digestive juices. One of the most important juices it makes is insulin. The insulin passes into the blood stream where it controls the amount of sugar in your body.

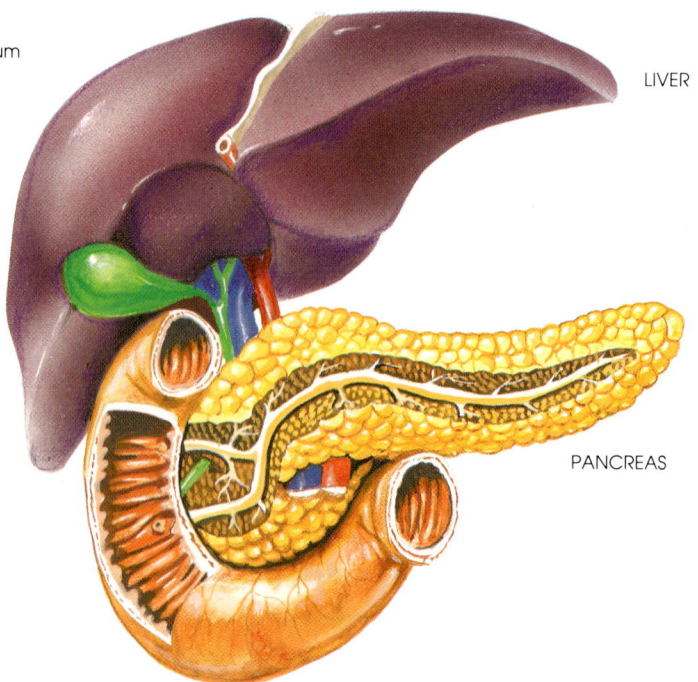

LIVER

PANCREAS

Did you know?

Nobody really knows what your appendix (a small, worm-shaped organ which lies where your small and large intestine meet) actually does! Some scientists think it may make white blood cells which fight germs in the intestines, but no-one is quite certain.

How large is my small intestine?

About four times as long as your body and between two and four centimetres wide, depending on how big you are. Your small intestine is coiled and folded to fit inside your belly. The first part is called the duodenum. It receives partly digested food from your stomach which, with the help of bile from your gall bladder and digestive juices from your pancreas, is broken down still further.

And how small is my large intestine?

Your large intestine shouldn't really be called 'large'. It is shorter than the small intestine – about as long as your body – and in some parts it is even narrower than the small intestine, although in other parts it is wider. Its function is to absorb water from the remaining material in your gut. As this happens, the material becomes drier and more solid until it forms faeces. Faeces are stored in the last part of the large intestine, the rectum, and leave the body through an opening called the anus.

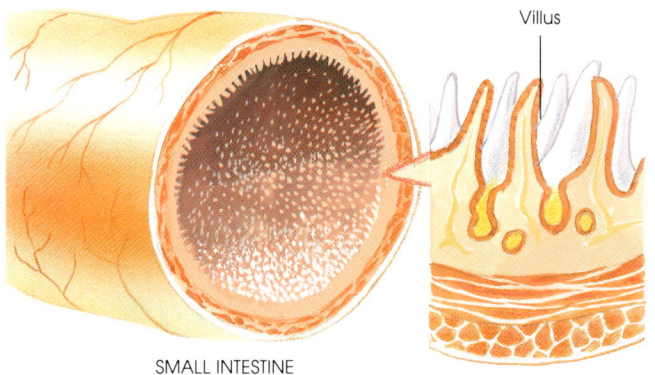

Villus

SMALL INTESTINE

LARGE INTESTINE   SMALL INTESTINE

Appendix

RECTUM

Is my small intestine really lined with velvet?

No, but it certainly looks like it. The inner lining of this intestine is folded and crumpled to make its surface area as big as possible. It is also lined with millions of tiny 'fingers' called villi supplied with blood vessels. Each villus, in turn, has even tinier 'fingers' called microvilli. These 'fingers' give it a velvety appearance. As food moves along your small intestine it is churned about and broken down by digestive juices. Food that has been broken down into small enough parts passes into the villi and is sent to your liver from where your blood takes it to the different parts of your body.

Where does urine come from?

Urine is made in the kidneys. These bean-shaped organs lie on either side of your body, just above your waist. Blood containing waste matter enters each kidney through a large artery. Tiny filters in the outer part of each kidney sift impurities and poisons from the blood. The impurities then travel through tiny tubes to the middle part of your kidney where they form a straw-coloured liquid called urine. The urine passes into a large tube called the ureter which leads to your bladder. The bladder stores the urine which passes out of your body when you go to the toilet.

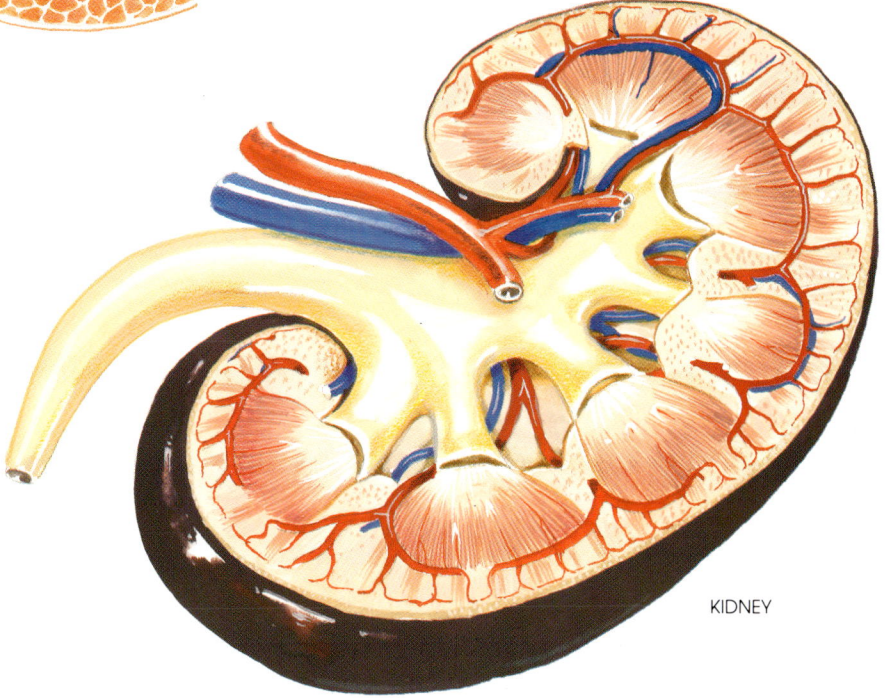

KIDNEY

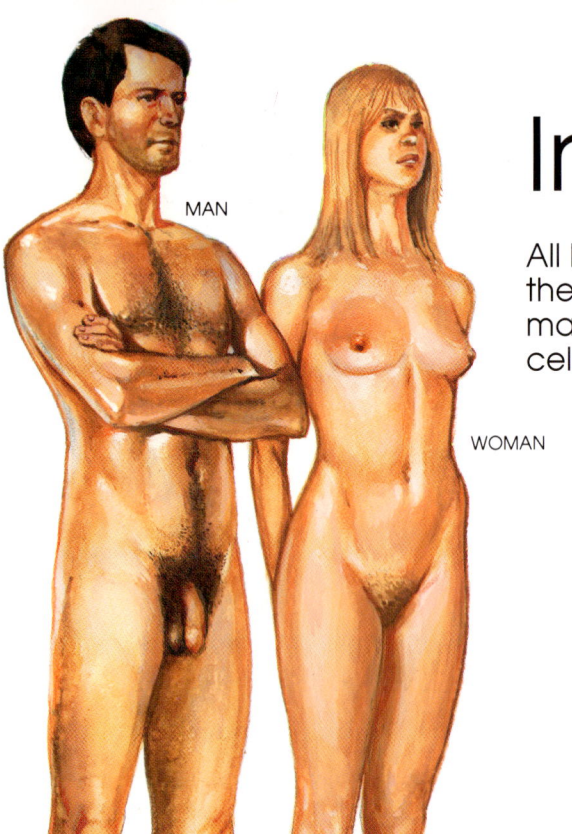

MAN

WOMAN

In the beginning

All living beings produce other living beings just like themselves. We say that they reproduce. When a man's sperm cell joins with a woman's female egg cell, a new life is created.

When do I stop being a child?

You don't suddenly change from a child into an adult. The change is gradual and usually begins between the ages of about 11 and 15, a stage known as adolescence or puberty. During this time a gland in your brain makes large amounts of sex hormones which cause changes in your body. In girls, breasts begin to bud, hips grow wider and waists become slimmer, menstruation starts and hair grows in the pubic area and under the arms. Boys also grow hair in the pubic area and under the arms. Beards and moustaches begin to sprout, and voices break. Girls and boys grow very quickly during the years of adolescence.

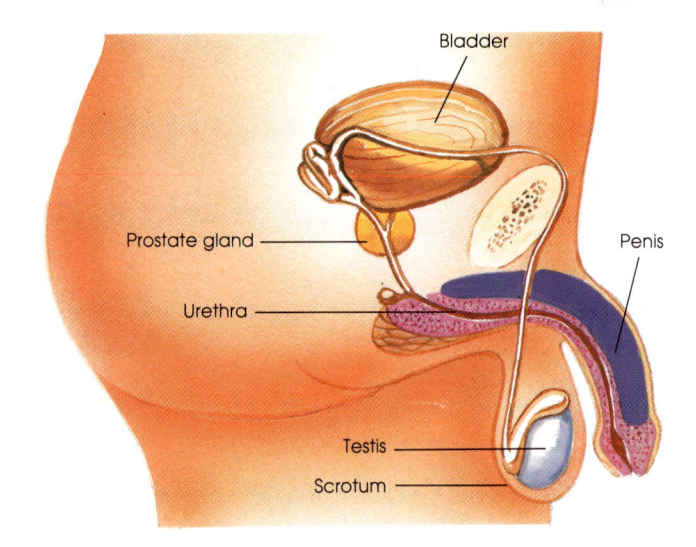

MALE REPRODUCTIVE SYSTEM

How much sperm does a boy's body make?

A boy's testicles start to make sperm at puberty. By the age of about 15 they make about 200 million sperm cells a day. A grown man's testicles make about 300 million sperm cells a day. The sperm is stored in a coiled tube called the epididymis inside the scrotum. If it is not used, the sperm cells die and are absorbed into the body.

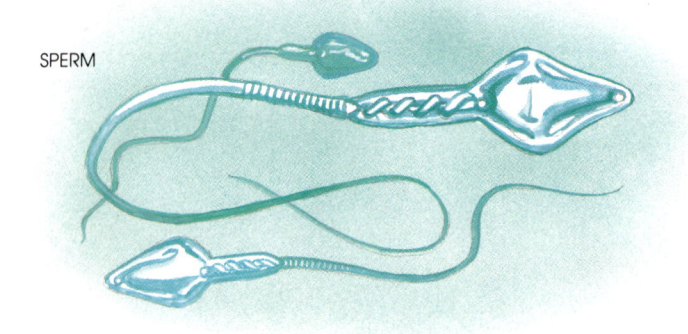

SPERM

Why are a man's sexual organs outside his body?

Men have two sexual organs outside the body: two ball-shaped testicles, which make sex cells called sperm, and a penis, used to place sperm inside a woman. The testicles need cool surroundings to do their work properly, and so they hang outside the body in a bag of skin called the scrotum. But men have sexual organs inside their bodies too. The seminal vesicle and the prostate gland, for example, make a milky fluid which helps sperm flow through the penis. This fluid, containing sperm, is called semen.

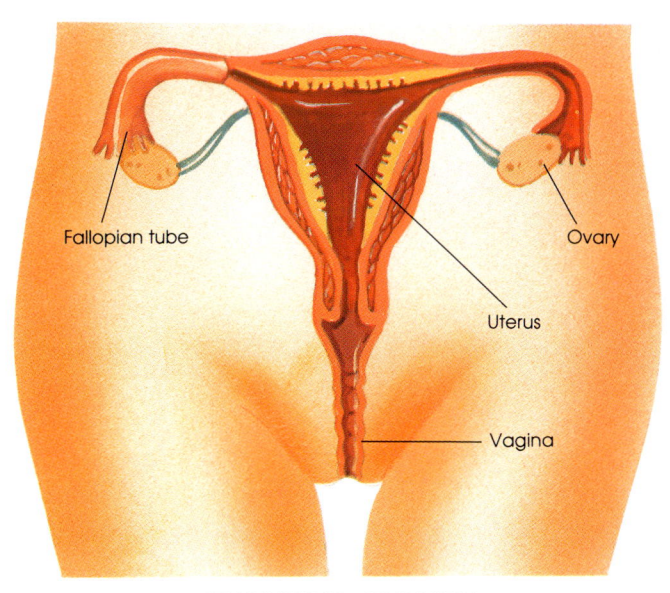

FEMALE REPRODUCTIVE SYSTEM

Fallopian tube

Ovary

Uterus

Vagina

Why are a woman's sexual organs mostly inside her body?

For protection. A woman's reproductive parts do many things: they make eggs called ova, they receive sperm cells from a man through his penis and they provide a place for a baby to develop. Inside her body are the ovaries (which make ova) and the parts that receive sperm cells. These include a tube called the vagina and a cavity called the womb, or uterus, where a baby develops. The parts outside her body are the breasts, which are used to feed a baby, and the vulva, the area between the legs into which the man's penis is placed.

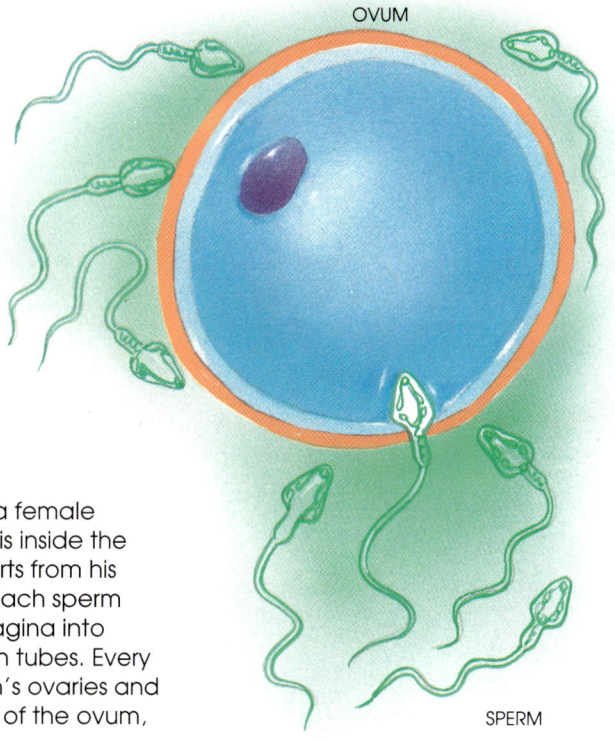

OVUM

SPERM

Why do women menstruate?

Every month, the lining of a woman's uterus becomes thick and rich in blood to provide a snug place for a fertilised egg to grow. If the egg is not fertilised, the egg and the lining are flushed out of the uterus through the vagina. This process is called a menstrual period.

How are babies made?

A baby is formed or conceived when a sperm cell joins with a female egg cell. This may happen when the man gently puts his penis inside the woman's vagina and moves it up and down until semen squirts from his penis into her vagina. We say that the man has ejaculated. Each sperm cell looks rather like a tadpole. It uses its tail to swim up the vagina into the womb, and then finally into two tubes called the fallopian tubes. Every month a single egg, or ovum, bursts out of one of the woman's ovaries and moves into the fallopian tube. If a sperm cell pierces the wall of the ovum, we call this fertilisation, or conception.

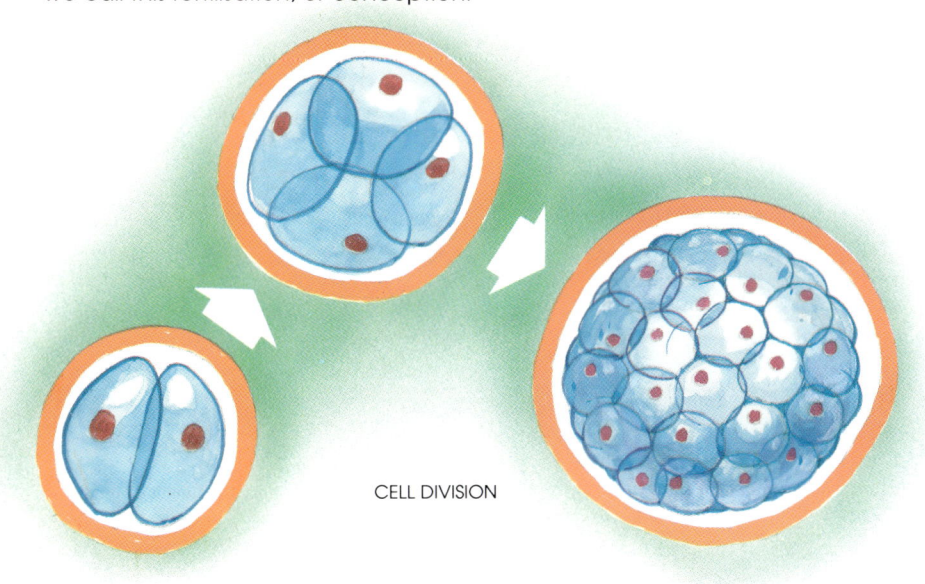

CELL DIVISION

What did I look like in my first few days of life?

You were just a ball of cells. A few hours after an ovum is fertilised, it begins to divide and grow. First it splits into two halves. Then each half splits so that there are four cells. Then each of these splits to make eight. After about five or six days of dividing and getting bigger, the ovum moves down the fallopian tube and into the womb, where it burrows into the thick, nutritious lining and grows and develops further. About nine months later a baby is born.

Index

Answers
1. Brain
2. Lungs
3. Heart
4. Skull
5. Stomach
6. Kidney